F. A. Davis Company

Always at your side...

IV Med Notes

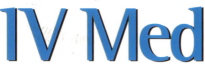

Nurse's Clinical Pocket Guide

D0219639

Gladdi Tomlinson
Deborah A. Ennis

Wipe-Free and Reusable

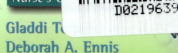

Includes...

- ✔ Wipe-Free Forms
- ✔ Administering IV Meds
- ✔ Top 200 Commonly Administered Meds
- ✔ IV Compatibilities with 50 Commonly Used Drugs
- ✔ IV Compatibilities with Potassium
- ✔ IV Compatibilities with Solutions
- ✔ Common Calculations
- ✔ Flushing IV Lines
- ✔ Common IV Complications
- ✔ Rate of Drug Administration

Abbreviations/Definitions

Admix: Adding a medication to another medication or solution

Bolus: A large amount of medication administered rapidly intravenously for therapeutic or diagnostic purposes

Compatibility: The ability of two or more drugs to be given concurrently without producing an undesirable effect; for example, if incompatible drugs are given together, that may produce a precipitate and create harmful effects to the patient

Continuous Infusion: An infusion usually given over at least 24 hours

Direct IV: IV push

Further Dilute: Add the mixture to a piggyback bag

Infusion: Administering a fluid, medication, or electrolyte into a vein

Intermittent Infusion: An infusion given via piggyback (IVPB)

IVP (IV Push): Usually given in the port closest to the patient

IVPB (IV Piggyback): Usually given in the port closest to the IV bag

Lumen: An IV catheter that can be used to inject or withdraw fluids; for example, a triple-lumen IV catheter is an IV catheter with three different lumens (see Tab 1 for an illustration)

Y-site: A port on intravenous tubing for the purpose of medication administration

Contacts • Phone/E-Mail

Name:	
Ph:	e-mail:

Name:	
Ph:	e-mail:

Name:	
Ph:	e-mail:

Name:	
Ph:	e-mail:

IV MED
Notes

Nurse's Clinical Pocket Guide

Gladdi Tomlinson, RN, MSN
Deborah A. Ennis, RN, MSN, CCRN

Purchase additional copies of this book
at your health science bookstore or
directly from F. A. Davis by shopping
online at www.fadavis.com or by calling
800-323-3555 (US) or 800-665-1148 (CAN)

A Davis's Notes Book

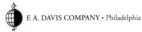

F. A. DAVIS COMPANY · Philadelphia

F.A. Davis Company
1915 Arch Street
Philadelphia, PA 19103
www.fadavis.com

Copyright © 2006 by F.A. Davis Company

All rights reserved. This book is protected by copyright. No part of it may be reproduced, stored in a retrieval system, or transmitted in any form or by any means, electronic, mechanical, photocopying, recording, or otherwise, without written permission from the publisher.

Printed in China by Imago

Last digit indicates print number: 10 9 8 7 6 5 4 3 2 1

Publisher, Nursing: Joanne Patzek DaCunha, RN, MSN
Project Editor: Ilysa H. Richman
Content Developmental Manager: Darlene Pedersen
Consultants: Michele Bunning, RN, MSN; Ilene Borze, RN, MS
Manager of Art & Design: Carolyn O'Brien

As new scientific information becomes available through basic and clinical research, recommended treatments and drug therapies undergo changes. The author(s) and publisher have done everything possible to make this book accurate, up to date, and in accord with accepted standards at the time of publication. The authors, editors, and publisher are not responsible for errors or omissions or for consequences from application of the book, and make no warranty, expressed or implied, in regard to the contents of the book. Any practice described in this book should be applied by the reader in accordance with professional standards of care used in regard to the unique circumstances that may apply in each situation. The reader is advised always to check product information (package inserts) for changes and new information regarding dose and contraindications before administering any drug. Caution is especially urged when using new or infrequently ordered drugs.

ISBN-13: 9780-8036-1446-8
ISBN-10: 0-8036-1446-2

Authorization to photocopy items for internal or personal use, or the internal or personal use of specific clients, is granted by F.A. Davis Company for users registered with the Copyright Clearance Center (CCC) Transactional Reporting Service, provided that the fee of $.10 per copy is paid directly to CCC, 222 Rosewood Drive, Danvers, MA 01923. For those organizations that have been granted a photocopy license by CCC, a separate system of payment has been arranged. The fee code for users of the Transactional Reporting Service is: 8036-1446/06 0 + $.10.

Place 2 $\frac{7}{8}$ × 2 $\frac{7}{8}$ **Sticky Notes** here

For a convenient and refillable note pad

✓ **HIPAA Supportive**
✓ **OSHA Compliant**

Waterproof and Reusable
Wipe-Free Pages

Write directly onto any page of *IV Med Notes*
with a ballpoint pen. Wipe old entries off with
an alcohol pad and reuse.

ASSESS INTERACT CALC IV PUSH **IVPB** CRIT THINK MED COMPAT

Look for our other Davis's Notes titles

RNotes®: *Nurse's Clinical Pocket Guide, 2nd edition*
ISBN-10: 0-8036-1335-0 / ISBN-13: 978-0-8036-1335-5

Coding Notes: *Medical Insurance Pocket Guide*
ISBN-10: 0-8036-1493-4 / ISBN-13: 978-0-8036-1493-2

Derm Notes: *Dermatology Clinical Pocket Guide*
ISBN-10: 0-8036-1495-0 / ISBN-13: 978-0-8036-1495-6

ECG Notes: *Interpretation and Management Guide*
ISBN-10: 0-8036-1347-4 / ISBN-13: 978-0-8036-1347-8

IV Therapy Notes: *Nurse's Clinical Pocket Guide*
ISBN-10: 0-8036-1288-5 / ISBN-13: 978-0-8036-1288-4

LabNotes: *Guide to Lab and Diagnostic Tests*
ISBN-10: 0-8036-1265-6 / ISBN-13: 978-0-8036-1265-5

LPN Notes: *Nurse's Clinical Pocket Guide*
ISBN-10: 0-8036-1132-3 / ISBN-13: 978-0-8036-1132-0

MA Notes: *Medical Assistant's Pocket Guide*
ISBN-10: 0-8036-1281-8 / ISBN-13: 978-0-8036-1281-5

MedNotes: *Nurse's Pharmacology Pocket Guide*
ISBN-10: 0-8036-1109-9 / ISBN-13: 978-0-8036-1109-2
New edition coming Fall 2006

MedSurg Notes: *Nurse's Clinical Pocket Guide*
ISBN-10: 0-8036-1115-3 / ISBN-13: 978-0-8036-1115-3

NutriNotes: *Nutrition & Diet Therapy Pocket Guide*
ISBN-10: 0-8036-1114-5 / ISBN-13: 978-0-8036-1114-6

OB Peds Women's Health Notes: *Nurse's Clinical Pocket Guide*
ISBN-10: 0-8036-1466-7 / ISBN-13: 978-0-8036-1466-6

Ortho Notes: *Clinical Examination Pocket Guide*
ISBN-10: 0-8036-1350-4 / ISBN-13: 978-0-8036-1350-8

PsychNotes: *Clinical Pocket Guide*
ISBN-10: 0-8036-1286-9 / ISBN-13: 978-0-8036-1286-0

*For a complete list of Davis's Notes and
other titles for health care providers,
visit www.fadavis.com*

An assessment of all of the following must be done prior to preparing to give an intravenous (IV) medication.

IV Site Assessment

Redness/inflammation—Caused by increased blood flow to the site. This is the body's protective response to irritation or injury.

Swelling—Caused by infiltration of the IV solution flowing into the surrounding tissue. Can also be caused by inflammation/infection.

Tenderness—Caused by the inflammatory process and increased blood flow to the area.

Coolness—Usually accompanied with edema—due to decreasing blood supply to the area.

Warmness—Usually indicates inflammation/infection at the site.

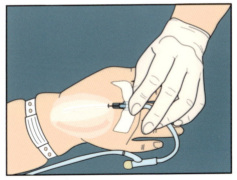

Infiltration—Occurs when IV fluids leak into the surrounding tissue around the venipuncture site. This is indicated by pain, swelling, coolness, and pallor around the site.

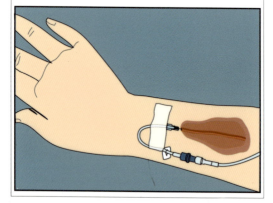

Phlebitis—Inflammation of the vein occurs from IV solutions and drugs and type and position of the IV catheter. Inflammation is manifested by pain, redness, edema, and warm skin temperature around the IV site.

Access Assessment

Peripheral

- Intermittent peripheral infusion device (IPID): Saline well, heparin well, heparin lock, or saline lock
- IV catheter to a continuously infusing IV line

Central

Single, double, triple, quad—lumen central line

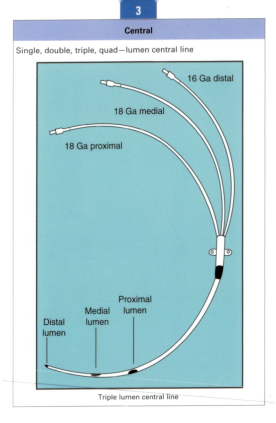

16 Ga distal

18 Ga medial

18 Ga proximal

Proximal lumen

Medial lumen

Distal lumen

Triple lumen central line

Each lumen has its own pathway (see following below) and its own exit. The medications never meet in the catheter, thus providing the ability to give incompatible medications. Due to the large volume of blood in the vessel, any infused medication is quickly dispersed.

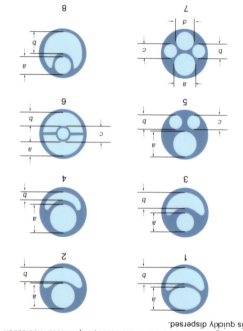

Cross-sectional view of multiple lumen central lines

■ Subcutaneous implanted vascular access port (also called Mediport)

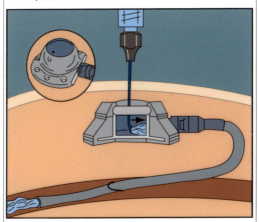

Mediport

Mediports are indicated for patients who require long-term treatment and are available in single- and double-injection ports. They are surgically implanted under the skin, with the catheter typically positioned in the superior vena cava. No part of the device can be seen outside the body.

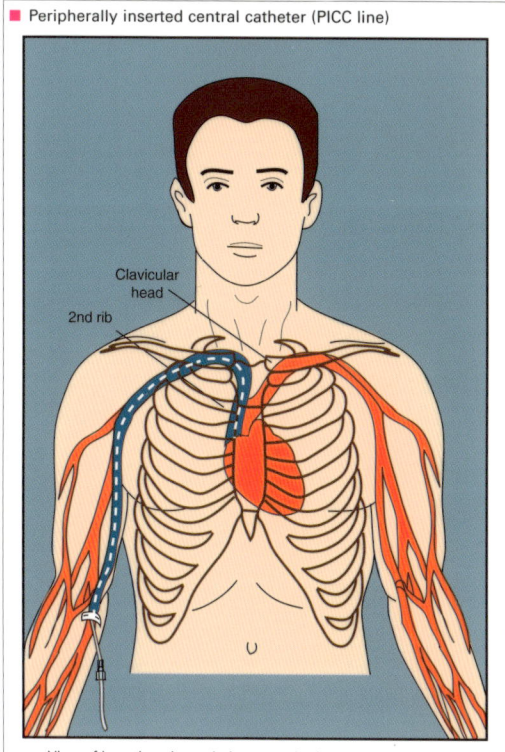

■ Peripherally inserted central catheter (PICC line)

Clavicular head

2nd rib

View of insertion site and placement in the superior vena cava

HOT TIP: When injecting medications or fluid via syringe into a PICC line, a syringe 10 cc or larger must be used to maintain a psi (pound per square inch) of nearly 7. A smaller syringe exerts too much psi, and the PICC catheter could burst.

Infusion Assessment

Primary infusion fluid—Fluid that is infusing continuously.

Secondary infusion—Fluid that is infusing intermittently, usually in a 50-250 ml IV bag infusing over 15 minutes to 2 hours.

Patient-controlled analgesia (PCA) pump—Infuses pain medication and is usually connected to the primary line. Both the primary line and PCA pump infuse concurrently.

HOT TIP: When assessing the infusions to check for incompatibilities, the PCA pump can easily be overlooked!! Verify the type of medication in the PCA pump, and ensure it is compatible.

Total parenteral nutrition (TPN)/Lipids—TPN usually infuses continuously over 24 hours. Lipids usually infuse over 8, 10, or 12 hours connected to the TPN IV line below the filter.

HOT TIP: Due to the additional components/medications in the TPN solution, NO medication is to be given in the same line as the TPN or the lipids.

Blood products—Include whole blood, packed red blood cells, plasma, platelets, albumin, serum globulins.

HOT TIP: NEVER give any medication in the blood component IV line. The only compatible solution is 0.9% normal saline.

Patient Identification

- Most facilities require two forms of identification (name, birth date, medical record number)
- Patient identification must be verified using the medication administration record and comparing it with the patient's identification band on each medication administration.

Syringe Types

Choose the correct syringes for medication administration according to the IV line and the amount of medication to be given. Some central IV lines require a 10 ml syringe.

Needle Types

- If your facility does not have the needleless or positive flow system, do not use a needle longer than 1 inch to put into the Y-site of a tubing. A longer-length needle could puncture the tubing.
- If your facility uses the positive flow valve system, you can leave the needle in place after preparation to carry it to the patient's room. Prior to administering the medication, remove the needle, and attach the syringe to the positive flow valve system.

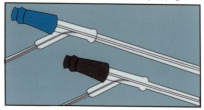

Positive flow valve system: no needle required

Laboratory Studies

Peak and Trough—Often ordered for patients receiving IV antibiotics. If a peak and trough is ordered, a blood level must be drawn prior to the antibiotic (trough); then the antibiotic is given, followed by another blood level (peak).

Drug level determinations/Serum levels—Monitors for toxicity/overdose. Ordered for patients receiving certain types of medications such as:

- potassium
- Digoxin (Lanoxin)
- Dilantin (phenytoin)
- Aminophylline
- Heparin and lovenox (PTT levels)

HOT TIP: Drug levels should be routinely monitored. Prior to administering medications that require serum levels, check the recent blood studies to determine if the medication should be given. Notify the physician in case of abnormal results to determine a change in medication dosage.

IV Solutions

Hypotonic Solutions (<250 mOsm/L)

Solution	Action	Indications	Nursing Interventions/Concerns
■ 2.5% dextrose in water solution ■ 0.25% sodium chloride solution ■ 0.33% sodium chloride solution ■ 0.45% sodium chloride solution	Will hydrate the cells; pulls fluid from the vascular space into the cellular space	Treatment of hypertonic dehydration	These solutions may further exaggerate hypotension due to fluid shifting out of vascular space; do not administer these solutions to hypotensive patients.

Isotonic Solutions (250-375 mOsm/L)

Solution	Action	Indications	Nursing Interventions/Concerns
■ 5% dextrose in water ■ 0.9% sodium chloride solution ■ Ringer's injection ■ Lactated Ringer's solution	Will hydrate the extracellular compartment; replaces fluid volume without disrupting the intracellular and interstitial volumes	Treatment of vascular dehydration; replaces sodium and chloride	5% dextrose in water is isotonic when infused but becomes hypotonic when the dextrose has been metabolized. Use cautiously in patients who are fluid-overloaded or who would be compromised if vascular volume would increase, such as renal and cardiac patients.

IV Solutions (Continued)

Hypertonic Solutions (>375 mOsm/L)

Solution	Action	Indications	Nursing Interventions/Concerns
■ 5% dextrose in 0.45% sodium chloride solution ■ 5% dextrose in 0.9% sodium chloride solution ■ 5% dextrose in lactated Ringer's solution ■ 10% dextrose in water ■ 20% dextrose in water ■ 50% dextrose in water ■ 70% dextrose in water	Will draw fluid out of intracellular space, leading to increased extracellular volume both in vascular and interstitial space	Treatment of hypotonic dehydration; treatment of circulatory collapse; increase fluid shift from interstitial space to vascular space	These solutions can be very irritating to veins, so observing the IV site for inflammation is imperative; may cause circulatory overload, so these solutions should be infused slowly to prevent this in vulnerable patients; may increase serum glucose in patients with glucose intolerance, which would make more frequent glucose monitoring an important nursing intervention

(Continued text on following page)

IV Solutions (Continued)

Hypertonic Solutions (>375 mOsm/L)

Solution	Action	Indications	Nursing Interventions/Concerns
■ 3% sodium chloride solution ■ 5% sodium chloride solution	Will draw fluid out of intracellular space, leading to increased extracellular volume both in vascular and interstitial space	Treatment of hypotonic dehydration; treatment of circulatory collapse; increase fluid shift from interstitial space to vascular space	These solutions can be very irritating to veins, so observing the IV site for inflammation is imperative; may cause circulatory overload, so these solutions should be infused slowly to prevent this in vulnerable patients; may increase serum glucose in patients with glucose intolerance, which would make more frequent glucose monitoring an important nursing intervention

Plasma Expanders

Solution	Action	Indications	Nursing Interventions/Concerns
■ Dextran 70 (isotonic) ■ Dextran 40 (isotonic) ■ 10% mannitol (hypertonic) ■ 20% mannitol (hypertonic) ■ 5% albumin ■ 25% albumin	Increases volume in the vascular space	Emergency treatment of shock due to fluid or blood loss	Monitor patients carefully for circulatory overload; monitor for hypersensitivity reactions; **medications should not be given with or added to these solutions**

IV Solutions (Continued)

Plasma Expanders

Solution	Action	Indications	Nursing Interventions/Concerns
■ 6% hetastarch in 0.9% sodium chloride ■ 10% hetastarch in 0.9% sodium chloride	Will draw fluid out of intracellular space, leading to increased extracellular volume both in vascular and interstitial space	Treatment of hypotonic dehydration; treatment of circulatory collapse; increase fluid shift from interstitial space to vascular space	These solutions can be very irritating to veins, so observing the IV site for inflammation is imperative; may cause circulatory overload, so these solutions should be infused slowly to prevent this in vulnerable patients; may increase serum glucose in patients with glucose intolerance, which would make more frequent glucose monitoring an important nursing intervention

Assessment

Patient Initials: _____ **Room #** _____

How does the IV site look?
_____ Without complications
_____ Redness
_____ Swelling
_____ Tenderness
_____ Coolness/Warmth
_____ Infiltration
_____ Phlebitis
_____ Comments:

Access Assessment:
Peripheral
_____ Location
_____ Central
_____ Location
_____ Type
_____ Type

Infusion Assessment:
Primary:
_____ Primary
_____ Tubing date:
Secondary:
_____ Tubing date:
Secondary:
_____ Tubing date:
_____ PCA pump:
Other comments:

Assessment

Patient Initials: _____   Room # _____

How does the IV site look?
_____ Without complications
_____ Redness
_____ Swelling
_____ Tenderness
_____ Coolness/Warmth
_____ Infiltration
_____ Phlebitis

Comments: _____
_____

Access Assessment:
_____ Peripheral
Location _____
Location _____
_____ Central
Type _____
Type _____

Infusion Assessment:
Primary: _____
Tubing date: _____
Primary: _____
Tubing date: _____
Secondary: _____
Tubing date: _____
Secondary: _____
Tubing date: _____
PCA pump: _____
Other comments: _____
_____
_____
_____
_____

Assessment

Patient Initials: _____ **Room #** _____

How does the IV site look?
Without complications _____
Redness _____
Swelling _____
Tenderness _____
Coolness/Warmth _____
Infiltration _____
Phlebitis _____
Comments: _____

Access Assessment:
Peripheral _____
Location _____
Central _____
Location _____
Type _____
Type _____

Infusion Assessment:
Primary _____
Tubing date: _____
Primary _____
Tubing date: _____
Secondary: _____
Tubing date: _____
Secondary: _____
Tubing date: _____
PCA pump: _____
Other comments: _____

Assessment

Patient Initials: _____   Room # _____

How does the IV site look?
_____ Without complications
_____ Redness
_____ Swelling
_____ Tenderness
_____ Coolness/Warmth
_____ Infiltration
_____ Phlebitis

Comments: _____
_____

Access Assessment:
_____ Peripheral
Location _____
Location _____
_____ Central
Type _____
Type _____

Infusion Assessment:
Primary: _____
Tubing date: _____
Primary: _____
Tubing date: _____
Secondary: _____
Tubing date: _____
Secondary: _____
Tubing date: _____
PCA pump: _____
Other comments: _____
_____
_____
_____
_____

When medication and solutions are combined to be infused intravenously, there can be undesirable effects. This tab discusses types of incompatibilities, administering medications with incompatible solutions, and pharmacokinetics.

Types of Incompatibilities

Physical—Occurs when a drug is mixed with another drug or solution in a syringe, IV tubing, or IV bag and results in an unsafe effect. This interaction creates a precipitate. This includes cloudiness, crystals, gas bubbles, or a precipitate that is not visible. For example: furosemide and ondansetron are not compatible and will create cloudiness in the syringe, tubing, or IV bag.

Chemical—Occurs when a drug is mixed with another drug or solution in a syringe, IV tubing, or IV bag and results in an alteration of drug potency. The most common form of a chemical incompatibility is the reaction between alkaline and acidic (pH) drugs or solutions. For example: some solutions that are very acidic, are dextrose. Many antibiotics are stable in dextrose for this reason; however, medications that are alkaline are unstable with dextrose. Therefore, it is better to combine alkaline solutions with normal saline. Solutions that are somewhat acidic or alkaline will not usually cause an infusion risk. But those that are not within the normal range may place the patient at risk for IV site phlebitis, fluid shift, or IV site irritation.

Therapeutic—Occurs when two or more drugs are being administered concurrently. This can produce either a decrease or increase in the therapeutic response. For example: if two antibiotics are given together or in sequence, one drug may antagonize the other and cause a therapeutic incompatibility. This incompatibility may be difficult to detect until the patient shows no clinical response to the drug.

HOT TIP: When checking drug compatibility, the source MUST list all drugs as compatible together. NEVER assume compatibility!

Administering Medications with Incompatible Solutions

- Acquiring assessment data prior to medication preparation is essential (see Tab 1). After determining what IV solutions/drugs are infusing, use a drug guide to research the drug compatibility of what is infusing into the patient.

HOT TIP: Make sure the IV tubing assessment includes any connections to other tubings For example: is there a PCA pump connected to the primary IV line? If so, the PCA drug must be included in the compatibility research!

- If incompatibility is determined, the line must be flushed with a compatible solution (most often, 0.9% normal saline) before and after administration of the drug (see Tab 5, IVPB, and Tab 6, Critical Thinking, for details).

Pharmacokinetics

Absorption—Rate at which the drug leaves the site of administration and enters the bloodstream or lymphatic system; also known as bioavailability. IV drugs are considered to be 100% bioavailable because they are given directly into the circulation. Absorption is affected by the physical and chemical properties of the drug, how the drug is manufactured, and the physiological characteristics of the patient.

Distribution—Actual transport of a drug in the body by the bloodstream. Rapid distribution occurs in the heart, liver, kidneys, and brain. Distribution is affected by circulatory status, total body fat, and solubility of the drug.

Metabolism (Biotransformation)—Process by which the body breaks down a drug and transforms it into an active chemical. The liver is the organ most responsible for metabolism. Metabolism is affected by disease conditions, other medications, and genetics.

Excretion—Process by which drugs are excreted by the body. The kidney is the organ most responsible for excretion. The liver and bowel also play an important role. Healthy kidney function is a key to excretion because of the glomerular filtration and tubular secretion.

Half-life—Time required for half of the drug to be removed from the body. Half-life is clinically important when determining blood levels of drugs such as Dilantin (phenytoin), aminophylline, and others.

Desired/Have × Quantity (Volume) Method

Physician's order
Penicillin G 1.5 million units every 4 hours

Have on hand
Penicillin G 200,000 units/ml

$$\frac{1,500,000 \text{ units} \times 1 \text{ ml}}{200,000 \text{ units}}$$

Get rid of unnecessary zeros

$$\frac{1,5\cancel{00,000} \text{ units} \times 1 \text{ ml}}{2\cancel{00,000} \text{ units}} = \frac{15}{2}$$

Units also cancel out because it occurs on both the top and the bottom of the equation. This means the answer will be in **ml**.

HOT TIP: Always multiply first, then divide. Remember <u>M</u>Y <u>D</u>EAR <u>A</u>UNT <u>S</u>ALLY Multiply, Divide, Add, Subtract

$$15 \times 1 = 15$$
$$15 \div 2 = \textbf{7.5 ml}$$

Ratio-Proportion Method

Physician's order
Penicillin G 1.5 million units every 4 hours

Have on hand
Penicillin G 200,000 units/ml

$$\frac{1,500,000 \text{ units}}{X} = \frac{200,000 \text{ units}}{1 \text{ ml}}$$

Cross-multiply:

1,500,000 units × 1 ml = 200,000 units X

1,500,000 units = 200,000 units X

Divide both sides by 200,000 to solve for X. Cancel out items that are the same on the top and the bottom.

$$\frac{1,500,000 \text{ unit} \quad ml}{200,000 \text{ units}} = \frac{200,000 \times}{200,000}$$

$$\frac{15 \text{ ml}}{2} = X$$

$$7.5 \text{ ml} = X$$

Drops per Minute:

$$\text{Formula} = \frac{ml \times \text{drop factor}}{\text{Time in minutes (not hours)}}$$

Have on hand

Infuse 150 ml over 1.5 hours

$$\frac{150 \text{ ml} \times 10 \text{ drops per min (gtt factor)}}{1.5 \text{ hr} \times 60 \text{ (to change to minutes)}}$$

HOT TIP: Drop factors can be found on the tubing packaging and in some instances on the tubing itself.

$$\frac{150 \text{ ml} \times 10 \text{ gtt/min} = 1500 \text{ gtt/min}}{1.5 \text{ hr} \times 60 \text{ min} = 75 \text{ min}}$$

$$\frac{1500 \text{ gtt/min}}{75 \text{ min}} = 20 \text{ gtt/min}$$

This same formula can work for an IVPB med:

$$\frac{50 \text{ ml} \times 10 \text{ gtt factor}}{30 \text{ min}} =$$

$$\frac{500}{30} = 16.66 = 17 \text{ gtt/min}$$

HOT TIP: When calculating gtt/min, the drop factor over time (in minutes) can easily be reduced to one number that you can then divide into the milliliters you wish to infuse to give you gtt/min as an answer.

For example:

$$\frac{50 \ \text{ml} \times \cancel{10} \ 1 \ \text{gtt/ml}}{\cancel{30} \ 3 \ \text{min}} = \frac{50 \times 1}{3} = \textbf{17 gtt/min}$$

$$\frac{50 \ \text{ml} \times \cancel{15} \ 1 \ \text{gtt/ml}}{\cancel{30} \ 2 \ \text{mins}} = \frac{50 \times 1}{2} = \textbf{25 gtt/min}$$

$$\frac{100 \ \text{ml} \times \cancel{10} \ 1 \ \text{gtt/ml}}{\cancel{60} \ 6 \ \text{min}} = \frac{100 \times 1}{6} = \textbf{17 gtt/min}$$

ml per Hour

Simply divide ml to infuse by the amount of time in hours to infuse.

Physician's order

1500 ml over 8 hours
1500/8 = 187.5 ml/hr or **188 ml/hr**

If using an infusion pump, set the pump to infuse fluid at this rate. If no infusion pump, use drops per minute formula. For example, a calculation with a drop factor of 10 is:

$$\frac{188 \times \cancel{10} \ (1)}{\cancel{60} \ (6)} = \frac{188}{6} = \textbf{31 gtt/min}$$

Calculating Drip Rates in ml/hr

Many medications are ordered as a continuous drip; for example, mg/hr or units/hr. The first two methods of drug calculations can be used to calculate the ml/hr for these drips. For example:

Physician's order: Lasix 20 mg/hr

Pharmacy sends Lasix 100 mg in 250 ml of 0.9% normal saline

Now use Desired/Have × Volume to solve for how many ml/hr to infuse this drip.

Calculating Drips for mcg/kg/min

Many critical care drips are administered by mg/kg/hr.

Desired/Have × Volume or Ratio-Proportion can assist this calculation as well.

1. Convert patient's weight to pounds if not already completed by dividing the pounds weight by 2.2.

$$\frac{55 \text{ lbs}}{2.2} = 25 \text{ kg}$$

Physician's order

2. Multiply the kg weight by the ordered medication dose.

Dopamine 5 mcg/kg/min

Have on hand

25 kg × 5 mcg = 125 mcg

Dopamine 400 mg/500 ml 5% dextrose and water

3. Convert the dopamine 400 mg to μg by multiplying by 1000. This can also be accomplished by moving the decimal point in the 400 by 3 places to the right. The solution is now 400,000 mcg/500 ml 5% dextrose and water.

4. Now place the numbers in the formula:

$$\frac{125 \text{ mcg (desired)} \times 500 \text{ ml (volume)}}{400,000 \text{ mcg (have on hand)}}$$

$$\frac{400,000}{125 \times 500} = \frac{400,000}{62,500} = \frac{400,000}{4000} = \frac{625}{4000} = 0.15625 \text{ ml/min}$$

HOT TIP: This method, as well as Ratio-Proportion, will work to calculate all drips when solving for ml/hr.

$$\frac{20 \text{ mg (desired)} \times 250 \text{ ml (volume)}}{100 \text{ mg (have on hand)}}$$

20 × 25 = 500

500/10 = **50 ml/hr**

5. To infuse this on an infusion pump, it is necessary to convert the ml/min to ml/hr. This is accomplished by multiplying the result by 60.

$$60 \times 0.15625 = 9.375 \text{ or } 9.4 \text{ ml/hr}$$

mg/kg

Physician's order

Nebcin 3.5 mg/kg/day in 2 equal doses every 12 hours.

Child's weight is 2 kg.

1. Multiply weight × dose

$$2 \text{ kg} \times 3.5 \text{ mg} = 7 \text{ mg/day}$$

2. Divide this dose by the number of times per day it is ordered to administer.

$$7 \text{ mg/2} = 3.5 \text{ mg for each dose given every 12 hours}$$

3. Calculate the amount of ml to give, using either Desired/Have × Volume or Ratio-Proportion.

Have on hand

Nebcin 0.5 mg/ml

$$\frac{3.5 \text{ mg (Desired)}}{0.5 \text{ mg (Have)}} \times 1 \text{ ml} = 7 \text{ ml given per dose}$$

Calculating Safe Dose

Used most often for pediatric doses

Physician's order

Penicillin V potassium 250 mg po every 8 hours

Manufacturer's stated safe dose range: 25-50 mg/kg/day

Have on hand

Penicillin V potassium 125 mg/5 ml

Child's weight = 45 pounds

1. Change the child's weight into kg.

   45/2.2 = 20.5 kg

2. Multiply the kg weight by each dose in the safe range to determine the safe range of medication per kg for this patient.

   20.5 × 25 = 512.5 mg/day
   20.5 × 50 = 1025 mg/day

3. Determine the total daily dose of medication the child is ordered.

   250 mg × 3 doses = 750 mg/day

4. Does the ordered dose fall within the safe doses that were calculated? In this situation, it does.

5. Now calculate how many ml to administer with each dose, using Desired/Have × Volume or Ratio-Proportion.

   $$\frac{250 \text{ mg}}{125 \text{ mg}} \times 5 \text{ ml} = 10 \text{ ml per dose}$$

Calculating Dose by Body Surface Area (BSA)

This method is also commonly used for pediatric doses:

Physician's order

Meperidine 30 mg/m²

Child's BSA: 1.0 m² (this can be determined using a nomogram)

Have on hand

Meperidine 25 mg/ml

1. Multiply the dose by the BSA

   30 mg × 1.0 m² = 30 mg (this is the desired dose)

2. Calculate one dose using Desired/Have × Volume or Ratio-Proportion.

   $$\frac{30 \text{ mg}}{25 \text{ mg}} \times 1 \text{ ml} = 1.2 \text{ ml}$$

Recommendations for Rounding

1. Infusion rates should be rounded to either a whole number
   or a whole number and one decimal point.
   For example: 30 ml/hr or 30.2 ml/hr
2. gtt/min should be rounded to a whole number.
   For example: 25 gtt/min
3. kg of body weight should be rounded to the tenth.
   For example: 40.47 kg should be rounded to 40.5 kg
4. Calculated dosages greater than 1 should be rounded to the
   tenth.
   For example: 1.666 ml should be rounded to 1.7
5. Calculated dosages less than 1 should be rounded to the
   hundredth.
   For example: 0.457 ml should be rounded to 0.46 ml

Phillips LD. IV Therapy Notes: Nurse's Clinical Pocket Guide. FA Davis
Company. Philadelphia. 2004.)

IV Fluid Rates in Drops per Minute

Rate ml/hr →	TKO	50	75	100	125	150	175	200	250
10 gtt/ml set	5	8	13	17	21	25	29	33	42
12 gtt/ml set	6	10	15	20	25	30	35	40	50
15 gtt/ml set	8	13	19	25	31	37	44	50	62
20 gtt/ml set	10	17	25	33	42	50	58	67	83
60 gtt/ml set	30	50	75	100	125	150	175	200	250

Note: TKO is 30 ml/hr.
Myers E. RNotes: Nurse's Clinical Pocket Guide, 2nd ed. FA Davis
Company. Philadelphia, 2006.

There are two acceptable methods of injecting medications directly into a patient, also known as the IV push methods. This section discusses both these methods.

Administering IV Push Medication: I

This section discusses administering IV push medication into a continuously infusing IV line:

- The first step requires completing all the assessment steps listed in Tab 1.
- Prepare the medication for injection as directed by your hospital's policy and/or by the manufacturer's recommendations.
- Ensure that the primary IV line is infusing at approximately 100 ml/hr. This ensures that the medication infuses quickly and that you achieve a quick response to the medication.
- If the patient's IV is infusing at a slower rate, then increasing the rate for a short period to administer the medication is usually not a problem.

HOT TIP: Never increase the IV rate of a primary line if there is medication in the primary IV solution such as potassium chloride or heparin.

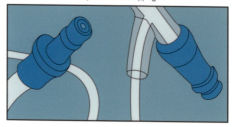

Positive pressure valve

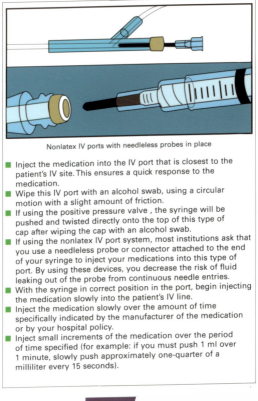

Nonlatex IV ports with needleless probes in place

- Inject the medication into the IV port that is closest to the patient's IV site. This ensures a quick response to the medication.
- Wipe this IV port with an alcohol swab, using a circular motion with a slight amount of friction.
- If using the positive pressure valve , the syringe will be pushed and twisted directly onto the top of this type of cap after wiping the cap with an alcohol swab.
- If using the nonlatex IV port system, most institutions ask that you use a needleless probe or connector attached to the end of your syringe to inject your medications into this type of port. By using these devices, you decrease the risk of fluid leaking out of the probe from continuous needle entries.
- With the syringe in correct position in the port, begin injecting the medication slowly into the patient's IV line.
- Inject the medication slowly over the amount of time specifically indicated by the manufacturer of the medication or by your hospital policy.
- Inject small increments of the medication over the period of time specified (for example: if you must push 1 ml over 1 minute, slowly push approximately one-quarter of a milliliter every 15 seconds).

IV PUSH

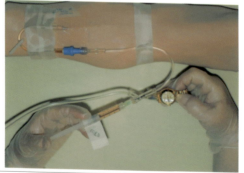

■ As you are injecting the medication into the IV line, it is correct to pinch the tubing of the IV line each time you inject medication into the line. It is also correct to not pinch the tubing, but instead slowly inject the medication into the port, with the IV continuing to infuse. Consider these issues, and decide whether you wish to pinch the tubing or not:

■ If you pinch the tubing, you will be giving your patient a small bolus of medication every time you inject medication.

■ If you pinch the tubing and your IV line is on an infusion pump, the pump will alarm due to high pressure in the line.

■ By not pinching, your medication will be quickly diluted by the IV solution and then be less irritating to the vein.

■ Concern arises about medication possibly moving backward into the line, as opposed to moving forward into the vein if you do not pinch; however, if you have a running IV, even if a small amount of medication moves backward in the line, then the flow of fluid will push the medication forward into the patient's vein.

■ It is your choice to either pinch the tubing or not. Both methods are correct.

30

PUSH

- Watch the IV line below the level of your port carefully during administration for the presence of crystals or milky type solutions in the tubing. This could indicate that there is an incompatibility in the line.
- If you do see crystals or milky type of fluids in the line, stop injecting the medication immediately.
- Clamp the tubing below the level of the crystals or milky solution. A hemostat works well for this, or fold the tubing in half to stop the IV flow, and ask another nurse to help you.
- Remove the IV line from the patient's site as quickly as possible, and flush the particulate matter out of the line.
- It is wise to change the tubing after a significant incompatibility situation.
- Crystals or precipitate material may act as embolic material if allowed to enter the patient's vascular system.
- Following administration of the medication, monitor your patient for the response that you are anticipating and also for adverse reactions to the medication.
- Document the medication as per your hospital's policy.

Administering IV Push Medication: II

Administering an IV push medication into an intermittent peripheral infusion device (IPID, saline well)—there are two methods:

- The first method uses saline flushes before and after the medication is injected directly into the IPID.
  - After following all the assessment steps in Tab 1, prepare three syringes.
    - Two syringes will contain 2-3 ml of normal saline solution.
    - The third syringe will contain the medication you have prepared to administer.

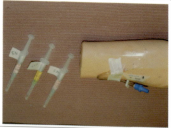

- Label each syringe with what you have placed in the syringe. A small piece of tape works very well and can be written on easily with a ballpoint pen.
- Line up the syringes near your patient in the order in which you intend to inject them.
- Wipe the port of the IPID with an alcohol swab.
- Insert the syringe into the port of the IPID containing saline and slowly inject the saline over 30 seconds. If you meet any resistance, you may need to restart the IPID. While injecting the saline, observe the site for signs of complications.

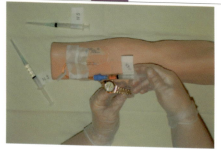

- Next, wipe the port again with the alcohol swab sitting at the port site; insert the syringe containing the medication, and infuse at the rate indicated by the manufacturer or by hospital policy.
- Next, again wipe the port with the alcohol swab; insert the second syringe containing the saline. Inject the first milliliter of saline over at least 1 minute. This prevents a bolus of medication from being injected into the patient's vein from the IPID cap. The second milliliter of saline can be infused over 30 seconds.

HOT TIP: REMEMBER—this administration method will produce almost immediate results from the medication. Watch your patient carefully for adverse reactions after administration.

- Document the medication as per your hospital protocol
- The second method entails using a 100-250 ml flush bag (normal saline or 5% dextrose and water) attached to primary IV tubing or infusion pump tubing and then attached to the cap of the IPID. This method produces running IV solution into the IPID, either by means of gravity or an infusion pump.

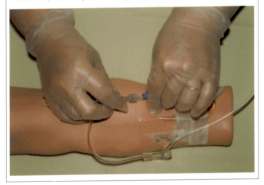

- Once you have inserted the end of the IV tubing into the IPID, allow the fluid to infuse for approximately 2 minutes at a rate of at least 100 ml/hr. If there is any resistance to flow, it may be necessary to restart the IPID.
- After 2 minutes have lapsed, you can then inject the medication into the port closest to the patient's IPID just as if injecting into a continuously infusing IV line.
- When you have completed injecting the medication, once again allow the IV flush to infuse for 2 minutes. This ensures that all the medication has been infused into the vein.
- After the 2 minutes have lapsed, disconnect the IV line from the IPID, place a sterile cover over the end of the tubing, and hang the tubing over the IV pole so it is ready for the next time medications need to be administered by this route. Most institutions require a final flush of 2–3 ml of saline to maintain patency of the saline well.
- This administration method elicits such a rapid response that you must evaluate your patient after administration for adverse reactions as well as for the response from the medication you anticipate.
- Document the medication as per your hospital protocol.

Piggyback (PB) medications can be administered through a continuous primary line or a flush bag Y-site. This tab discusses both methods.

Continuous Primary Line

Administering an IVPB medication into a continuously infusing IV solution:

- The first step is to complete all the assessment steps in Tab 1.
- Prepare the medication for infusion as directed by your facility's policy or by the manufacturer's recommendations.

Gravity Infusion

- Remove the secondary tubing from the package, and clamp the tubing immediately.
- Connect the piggyback bag to the secondary tubing, fill the chamber half full, and prime the tubing.
- Hang the IVPB bag on the IV pole.
- Using an alcohol wipe, wipe off the highest tubing Y-site port of the primary line.
- Insert the end of the IVPB tubing into this Y-site port.

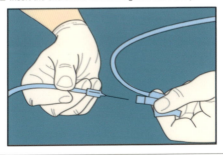

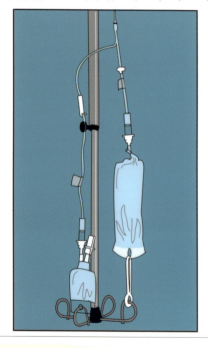

- Lower the primary bag with the hanger provided in the secondary tubing package.
- The IVPB bag should be in the highest position.

- Open the entire clamp of the IVPB bag.
- Control the medication's gtt/min with the primary tubing clamp.
- Once the medication begins to infuse, watch the IV line below the level of the port for the presence of crystals or a milky substance. This could indicate an incompatibility in the line and must be stopped immediately.

HOT TIP: After 10 minutes, check the patient and IV site for any reactions. If there is a reaction, turn off the medication, and notify the physician. Also, flush the medication out of the line.

After the IVPB infusion is complete, return the rate of the primary infusion back to its original rate.

Leave the IVPB bag in place to be used for the next dose of the same medication.

Electronic Infusion Pump

- Remove the secondary tubing from the package, and clamp the tubing immediately.
- Some pumps will require the primary bag to be lowered; check the pump instructions.
- Hang the IVPB bag on the IV pole.
- Lower the primary bag, if necessary, with the hanger provided with the secondary tubing package.
- Using an alcohol wipe, wipe off the highest tubing Y-site port of the primary line. On a pump, this port may be located where the primary tubing is inserted into the pump.
- Insert the end of the IVPB tubing into this port.
- Open the entire clamp of the IVPB bag.

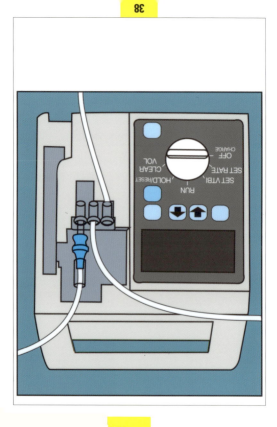

- Set the pump to infuse the IVPB bag by setting the volume and the rate; note the rate the primary bag is infusing in case you need to reset it after the completion of the IVPB.
- Once the medication begins to infuse, watch the IV line below the level of the connection port for the presence of crystals or a milky substance. This could indicate an incompatibility in the line and must be stopped immediately.

HOT TIP: After 10 minutes, check the patient and IV site for any reactions. If there is a reaction, turn off the medication, and notify the physician. Also, flush the medication out of the line.

After the IVPB infusion is complete, make sure the primary infusion is infusing at the original rate.

Leave the IVPB bag in place to be used for the next dose of the same medication.

Flush Bag (Normal Saline or D$_5$W):

- The first step is to complete all the assessment steps in Tab 1.
- Prepare the medication for infusion as directed by your facility's policy or by the manufacturer's recommendations.
- Wipe off the port of the patient's IV site with an alcohol wipe.
- Connect the flush bag line to the patient's IV site.
- Lower the flush bag.
- Set the flush bag to infuse at 100 ml/hr. Use the tubing drop factor to calculate gtt/min.
- Infuse the flush bag for 2 minutes.
- While the flush bag is infusing, set up the IVPB bag to the highest position.
- Using an alcohol wipe, wipe off the highest tubing Y-site port of the primary line.
- Insert the end of the IVPB tubing into this port.
- Open the entire clamp of the IVPB bag.
- Control the medication's gtt/min with the flush bag tubing clamp.

IVPB

- Once the medication begins to infuse, watch the IV line below the level of the connection port for the presence of crystals or a milky substance. This could indicate an incompatibility in the line and must be stopped immediately.
- After the IVPB infusion is completed, allow the flush bag to continue to infuse for 2-3 minutes to ensure the medication is out of the line.
- Disconnect the flush line from the patient's IV site.
- Place a sterile cap on the end of the flush bag tubing, and hang this tubing over the pole for another use.
- Flush the patient's IV site with 2-3 ml of an approved solution in a syringe—see your facility's policy. This is usually done with normal saline. Flush at a consistent rate.

How do I administer an IV push medication if my patient has a patient-controlled analgesia (PCA) pump?

- If you are giving a medication IV push into an infusing IV line that also has a PCA pump in line, first evaluate if the medication you wish to administer is compatible with the medication in the PCA pump. If it is compatible, then you may push the medication as described in Tab 4. If the medication is not compatible, you have **two options:**
  - Infuse the medication into another IV site, if one is available, or
  - Clamp your IV tubing just above the port closest to the patient's IV site, using a hemostat with the teeth covered to prevent cutting the IV tubing.
    - After clamping the line, inject 3-5 ml of sterile saline into the port.
    - Administer the IV push medication into that same port.
    - Inject another 3-5 ml of sterile saline into the port.
    - Unclamp your IV, and allow normal flow of the PCA and the patient's primary IV.
    - This method prevents the medication you wish to administer from coming in contact with the medication in the PCA pump.

How do I administer an IV push medication if my patient has a continuously infusing medication, such as heparin, Cardizem, or Lasix?

- If you are giving a medication IV push into an infusing IV line that also has a PCA pump in line, first evaluate if the medication you wish to administer is compatible with the medication in the PCA pump. If it is compatible, then you may push the medication as described in Tab 4.If the medication is not compatible, you have **two options:**
  - Infuse the medication into another IV site, if one is available, or
  - Clamp your IV tubing just above the port closest to the patient's IV site, using a hemostat with the teeth covered to prevent cutting the IV tubing.
    - After clamping the line, inject 3-5 ml of sterile saline into the port.

CRIT
THINK

- Administer the IV push medication into that same port.
- Inject another 3–5 ml of sterile saline into the port.
- Unclamp your IV, and allow normal flow of the patient's IV fluids and medications.
  - This method prevents the medication from coming in contact with the medication in the drip.

How do I administer an IVPB medication if my patient has a PCA pump?

■ If the medication you wish to infuse by IVPB is compatible with the PCA pump medication, you can administer the medication as previously described in Tab 4. If the medication is not compatible with the medication in the PCA pump, you have **two options**:

■ You can start another IV site, create an IPLD, and use that site to infuse any IVPB medications you may have.

■ If you cannot or do not wish to start a second line, and your medication is not compatible with the PCA then the only option is to:
- Have the patient push the PCA dose button just before starting the medication.
- Place the PCA in the off position. After the PCA is stopped, flush the line with 2–3 ml of solution compatible with the medication prior to starting the IVPB line.
- Start the IVPB medication, and infuse over the shortest time permitted by the manufacturer.
- After the IVPB medication has infused, allow 2 minutes for the primary IV line to fully flush with the primary solution, preventing interaction between the PCA medication and the IVPB medication.
- Return the PCA pump to operational level.

How do I administer an IVPB medication with a continuously infusing medication such as heparin, Cardizem, or Lasix?

■ If the medication you wish to infuse by IVPB is compatible with the continuously infusing medication, see Tab 4, providing the continuously infusing medication can be interrupted for the period of time that it will take to infuse the IVPB medication.

- If you cannot interrupt the continuously infusing medication for that period of time, **you must start a second IV site**.
- If the IVPB is not compatible with the continuously infusing medication but can be interrupted for the time it will take to infuse the IVPB, your option is:
  - Prepare a flush bag (250 ml of 0.9% sodium chloride solution or 5% dextrose and water) with primary tubing.
  - Attach the flush bag to the port closest to the patient's IV line. Start the flush bag infusing, and clamp off the continuously infusing medication with a hemostat, with the teeth covered.
  - If using a pump to infuse the medication, turn it off at this time.
  - Begin the IVPB medication through the flush line, and infuse at the fastest rate permitted by the manufacturer.
  - Allow the flush bag to continue to flush for 2 minutes after the IVPB medication has completed.
  - Discontinue the flush bag.
  - Unclamp the continuously infusing medication, and restart at the prescribed rate.
- If the IVPB is not compatible with the continuously infusing medication and that medication cannot be interrupted, start a second IV line to administer the IVPB medication.

How do I administer an IV push medication into solution that is not compatible with the medication?

- There are two options:
  - Option 1: While clamping the primary solution either by your hand or with a hemostat (with teeth covered), instill 3-5 ml of sterile saline into the port closest to the patient's IV site.
  - Follow this first flush with the medication, keeping the line clamped.
  - Follow the medication with another 3–5 ml of sterile saline flush.
  - Unclamp the line, and allow the primary solution to flow again.
  - Option 2: Attach a flush bag (250 ml of 0.9% sodium chloride solution or 5% dextrose and water) to the port closest to the patient's IV site. Clamp off the primary solution using previously stated methods.
  - Allow the flush to infuse for 2 minutes before and after the medication is injected.

CRIT THINK

- Disconnect the flush bag.
- Unclamp the primary solution and allow the solution to flow at the ordered rate.

How do I administer an IVPB into a solution that is incompatible with the IVPB medication?

You have two options:

- Option 1: Use another access site, and infuse the IVPB into the alternate access site.
- Option 2: Attach a flush bag (250 ml of 0.9% sodium chloride solution or 5% dextrose and water) to the port closest to the patient's IV site. Clamp off the primary solution using previously stated methods.
- Administer the IVPB through the flush bag.
- Allow the flush to infuse for 2 minutes before and after the medication is infused.
- Disconnect the flush bag.
- Unclamp the primary solution and allow the solution to flow at the ordered rate.

Why won't the IVPB infuse?

Check the following:

- Is the IV access patent?
- Is the tubing kinked in any place?
- Is the IVPB positioned higher than the primary solution?
- Has the clamp to the secondary tubing been opened fully?
- Are there any clamps on the tubing that are in the fully clamped position?

Why can't the medication be pushed into a patient's IV or IPID?

Check the following:

- Is the IV or IPID patent?
- Is there a clamp on any access areas or tubing that is in the fully clamped position?
- Is the tubing kinked in any place?

Can the patient's IV be increased to 100–125 ml/hr while the IV push medication is being administered?

- Yes, if there is no medication added to the primary solution.
- No, if there are medications added to the primary solution that cannot be infused at a higher rate (i.e., potassium chloride, heparin).

Flushing Intravenous Access Catheters

Access type	Flushing Solution	Solution Strength	Flushing Frequency
Peripheral Catheters			
Intermittent peripheral infusion device (IPID)	Normal saline	0.9% NaCl	2–3 ml every 12 hours and after every use
IPID—24 gauge or smaller	Heparin solution	10 units/ml	1 ml every 8 hours and after every use
Central Venous Catheters			
Midline catheter (non-Groshong)	Normal saline; heparin solution	0.9% NaCl 100 units/ml	2 ml normal saline followed by 2 ml of heparin solution to each lumen every 12 hours and after every use
Midline catheter (Groshong)	Normal saline	0.9% NaCl	2 ml normal saline every 12 hours to each lumen and after every use
Central Venous Catheters			
PICC (non-Groshong)	Heparin solution	100 units/ml	2 ml normal saline followed by 2 ml of heparin solution to each lumen every 12 hours and after each use

(Continued text on following page)

CRIT THINK

CRIT THINK

Access type	Flushing Solution	Solution Strength	Flushing Frequency
Central Venous Catheters			
PICC (Groshong)	Normal saline	0.9% NaCl	2 ml normal saline every 8-12 hours to each lumen and after every use
Central venous catheter (double, triple, and quadruple lumen) (without positive pressure cap device)	Normal saline; heparin solution	100 units/ml	2 ml normal saline followed by 2 ml of heparin solution every 24 hours to each lumen and after each use
Central Venous Catheters			
Central venous catheter (double, triple, and quadruple lumen) (with positive pressure cap device)	Normal saline	0.9% NaCl	2 ml normal saline every 24 hours to each lumen and after every use
Hickman & Broviac catheters (tunneled catheters) (without positive pressure cap device)	Normal saline; heparin solution	0.9% NaCl 100 units/ml	5 ml normal saline solution followed by 2-3 ml heparin solution every 24 hours to each lumen and after each use

(Continued text on following page)

Access type	Flushing Solution	Solution Strength	Flushing Frequency
Central Venous Catheters			
Hickman & Broviac catheters (tunneled catheters) (with positive pressure cap device)	Normal saline	0.9% NaCl	5 ml normal saline solution every 24 hours to each lumen and after each use
Implanted venous access devices (Mediport, Port-a-Cath) (accessed without positive pressure cap device)	Normal saline; heparin solution	0.9% NaCl 100 units/ml	5 ml normal saline solution followed by 5 ml heparin solution every 24 hours to each lumen and after each use
Implanted venous access devices (Mediport, Port-a-Cath) (accessed with positive pressure cap device)	Normal saline	0.9% NaCl	5 ml normal saline solution to each port every 24 hours and after each use

HOT TIP: Catheters with a valve tip, called Groshong catheters, DO NOT REQUIRE HEPARIN SOLUTION nor SHOULD THEY HAVE HEPARIN SOLUTION instilled through them!

HOT TIP: The above indicated flushing instructions are only guidelines. It is imperative that you follow your institution's policies for flushing these catheters!

CRIT THINK

Acyclovir (Zovirax)

- **Common Adult and Child (>12 yr) Dose:** 5–10 mg/kg every 8 hours for 5 days
- **Common Child Dose (<12 yr):** 10–20 ml/kg every 8 hours for 7–10 days
- **Reconstitution:** 500 mg vial with 10 ml of sterile water; 1 g vial with 20 ml of sterile water
- **Solution Amount:** 50 mg/ml
- **Compatible Solutions:** D₅W, D5/0.25% NaCl, D5/0.45% NaCl, D5/0.9% NaCl, 0.9% NaCl, lactated Ringer's (LR) solution
- **IV Push:** No
- **IVPB:** Yes
- **IV Infusion Time:** At least 60 minutes
- **Special Considerations:** Do not administer with blood products or any products containing protein; do not reconstitute with bacteriostatic solutions

Adenosine (Adenocard)

- **Common Adult and Child (>50 kg) Dose:** 6 mg; if no response, repeat in 1–2 minutes with 12 mg
- **Common Child Dose (<50 kg):** 0.05–0.1 mg/kg; may repeat in 1–2 minutes, increasing by 0.05–0.1 mg to a maximum dose of 0.3 mg/kg
- **Reconstitution:** No — give undiluted
- **Compatible Solutions:** All IV solutions
- **IV Push:** Yes
- **IV Push Rate:** Administer rapidly over 1–2 seconds. Slow administration will cause increased heart rate due to vasodilation
  - Must be administered as close to the IV site as possible
  - Follow infusion with a rapid saline flush to ensure medication reaches circulation before drug becomes inactive
  - Slow administration will cause increased heart rate due to vasodilation

- **IVPB:** Yes: administer 30 ml vial undiluted as a peripheral infusion
- **IVPB Infusion Rate:** 140 mcg/kg/min over 6 minutes for a total dose of 0.84 mg/kg. Thallium-201 should be injected as close to the venous access as possible at the midpoint (after 3 minutes) of the infusion
- **Special Considerations:** Following administration there may be a short period of first-, second-, or third-degree heart block or asystole; this will resolve quickly (in fewer than 12 seconds) due to the short duration of adenosine
- Patient must be on a cardiac monitor

Alatrofloxacin (Trovan)

- **Common Adult Dose:** 200–300 mg q 24 hours
- **Common Child Dose:** N/A
- **Reconstitution:** Create a concentration of 1–2 mg/ml
- **Solution Amount:** Create a concentration of 1–2 mg/ml
- **Compatible Solutions:** D₅W, D5/0.45% NaCl, D5/0.9% NaCl, 0.45% NaCl, 0.9% NaCl, D5/LR
- **IV Push:** No
- **IVPB:** Yes
- **IV Infusion Time:** 60 minutes
- **Special Considerations:** Discard unused portion

Albumin (Albuminar)

- **Common Adult Dose:** 500 ml of the 5% solution; may be repeated within 30 minutes (50–75 g of the 25% solution)
- **Common Child Dose:** 50 ml (infants and neonates: 10–20 ml/kg) of the 5% solution (25 g of the 25% solution)
- **Reconstitution:** 5% normal serum albumin should be administered undiluted; 25% normal serum albumin can be administered undiluted or diluted with 0.9% NaCl, D₅W, or sodium lactate solution
- **Solution Amount:** N/A

- **Compatible Solutions:** D_5W, D5/0.45% NaCl, D5/0.9% NaCl, 0.9% NaCl, LR, D5/LR, sodium lactate 1/6 M
- **IV Push:** No
- **IVPB:** Yes
- **IV Infusion Time:** Do not exceed 2–4 ml/min for 5% solutions; 1 ml/min for 25% solutions
- **Special Considerations:** Do not dilute with sterile water
- Solution should be clear and amber color

Alefacept (Amevive)

- **Common Adult Dose:** 7.5 mg once weekly for 12 weeks; after a 12-week rest period, a second course may be given
- **Reconstitution:** Use 0.6 ml of sterile water provided for a concentration of 7.5 mg/0.5 ml of alefacept; keep needle pointed toward the sidewall of the vial during reconstitution; inject diluent slowly, swirl gently; do not shake vigorously to avoid foaming; drug should dissolve in <2 minutes; solution should be clear and colorless to slightly yellow with no particulates
- **Compatible Solutions:** 0.9% NaCl
- **IV Push:** Yes
  - **IV Push Rate:** Administer over no longer than 5 seconds. Follow with 3.0 ml of 0.9% NaCl
  - Remove needle used for reconstitution, and replace with other needle provided
  - Prepare with two syringes with 3.0 ml of 0.9% NaCl to flush before and after injection; prime a winged infusion set with 3.0 ml of 0.9% NaCl, and insert into vein
- **IVPB:** No
- **Special Considerations:**
  - Administer immediately after reconstitution or within 4 hours if refrigerated
  - Do not filter administration
  - Do not mix with other diluents or medications
  - Discard unused medication 4 hours after reconstitution

Allopurinol (Zyloprim)

- **Common Adult Dose:** 200–600 mg/day in single or divided doses (q 6–12 hours)
- **Common Child Dose:** 200 mg/m^2/day as a single daily dose or in divided doses every 6–12 hours
- **Reconstitution:** Reconstitute a 30 ml vial with 25 ml of sterile water
- **Solution Amount:** Not greater than 6 mg/ml
- **Compatible Solutions:** 0.9% NaCl and D$_5$W
- **IV Push:** No
- **IVPB:** Yes
- **Infusion Time:** Not specified
- **Special Considerations:**
  - Must be administered within 10 hours after reconstitution
  - Do not refrigerate
  - Do not administer solutions that are discolored or that contain particulate matter

Alteplase (Activase)

- **Common Adult Dose:** *Myocardial Infarction (Accelerated):* 15 mg initially, then 0.75 mg/kg up to 50 mg over 30 minutes, then 0.5 mg/kg up to 35 mg over next 60 minutes. *Myocardial Infarction (Standard Regimen) Adults >65 kg:* 60 mg over 1st hour as a bolus over 1–2 minutes, 20 mg over the 2nd hour, and 20 mg over the 3rd hour for total dose of 100 mg. *Myocardial Infarction (Standard Regimen) Adults <65 kg:* 0.75 mg/kg over 1st hour given as a bolus over first 1–2 minutes, 0.25 mg/kg over the 2nd hour, and 0.25 mg/kg over the 3rd hour for a total dose of 1.25 mg/kg—not to exceed 100 mg total. *Pulmonary Embolism:* 100 mg over 2 hours followed by heparin. *Acute Ischemic Stroke:* 0.9 mg/kg given over 1 hour, with 10% of the dose given as a bolus over the 1st minute. *Occluded Venous Access Devices: (Adults and Children >30 kg):* 2 mg/2 ml instilled into occluded catheter; may repeat × 1

- **Common Child Dose:** *Occluded Venous Access Devices (10–30 kg):* 110% of lumen volume, not to exceed 2 mg/2 ml instilled into occluded catheter; may repeat once over 2 hours

- **Reconstitution:** Vials are packaged with sterile water for injection; do not use bacteriostatic water for injection; reconstitute 20 mg vials with 20 ml and 50 mg vials with an 18 gauge needle; avoid excess agitation during dilution; swirl or invert gently to mix; solution may foam upon reconstitution; bubbles will resolve upon standing for a few minutes

- **Solution Amount:** May be further diluted if desired immediately before use with equal amounts of fluid to solution

- **Compatible Solutions:** D_5W, 0.9% NaCl

- **IV Push:** Yes

- **IVPB:** Yes

- **IV Push Rate:** Bolus over 1 minute

- **IV Infusion Time:** 1–2 hours

- **Special Considerations:** Flush IV line with 20–30 ml of saline at completion of infusion to ensure entire dose is received

Amifostine (Ethyol)

- **Common Adult Dose:** 200 mg/m^2 15–30 minutes before radiation therapy; 910 mg/m^2 within 30 minutes before chemotherapy

- **Reconstitution:** Reconstitute a 500 mg vial with 9.7 ml of sterile 0.9% NaCl

- **Solution Amount:** 50 mg/ml

- **Compatible Solutions:** 0.9% NaCl

- **IV Push:** No

- **IVPB:** Yes

- **IV Infusion Time:** Administer over 15 minutes, 30 minutes before chemotherapy; administer over 3 minutes, 15–30 minutes before radiation therapy

- **Special Considerations:** Stable for 5 hours at room temperature and 24 hours if refrigerated; do not administer if solution is discolored or if it contains particulate matter

Amikacin (Amikin)

- **Common Adult Dose:** 5–7.5 mg/kg q 12 hours
- **Common Infant and Neonate Dose:** 10 mg/kg initially, then 7.5 mg/kg every 12 hours
- **Reconstitution:** N/A
- **Solution Amount:** 100–200 ml
- **Compatible Solutions:** D_5W, $D_{10}W$, 0.9% NS, D5/0.9% NaCl, D5/0.45% NaCl, D5/0.25% NaCl, LR
- **IV Push:** No
- **IVPB:** Yes
- **IV Infusion Time:** 30–60 minutes
- **Special Considerations:** Solution may be pale yellow without decreased potency
- Do not confuse with **Amicar**

Aminocaproic Acid (Amicar)

- **Common Adult Dose:** 4–5 g over 1st hour followed by 1 g/hr for 8 hours or until hemorrhage is controlled; 6 g over 24 hours after prostate surgery
- **Common Child Dose:** 50–100 mg/kg every 6 hours for 2–3 days for acute bleeding; or as a continuous infusion of 33.3 mg/kg/hr not to exceed 18 g/m²/24 hr
- **Reconstitution:** Dilute initial 4–5 g in 250 ml of sterile water for injection, 0.9% NaCl, D_5W, or LR (do not use sterile water in patients with subarachnoid hemorrhage); follow initial infusion with 1 g/hr diluted in 50–100 ml of solutions stated above
- **Solution Amount:** 4–5 g/250 ml of solution; 1 g in 50–100 ml of solution
- **Compatible Solutions:** 0.9% NaCl and D_5W, LR
- **IV Push:** No
- **IVPB:** Yes
- **Infusion Time:** Each dose over 1 hour
- **Special Considerations:**
  - Do not mix with any other medications

Aminophylline (Phyllocontin)

- **Common Adult and Child Dose (6 month old to adult):**
  Loading dose: 4.7 mg/kg, followed by an infusion of 0.55
  mg/kg/hr for 12 hours, followed by 0.36 mg/kg/hr
- **Common Child Dose:** 1–3 mg every 8–12 hours
- **Compatible Solutions:** D_5W, $D_{10}W$, $D_{20}W$, 0.9% NaCl, 0.45%
  NaCl, D5/0.9% NaCl, D5/0.45% NaCl, D5/0.25% NaCl, LR
- **IV Push:** No
- **IVPB:** Yes
- **IV Infusion Time:** Loading dose should be infused over 20–30
  minutes; longer infusions should not exceed 20–25 mg/min
- **Special Considerations:**
  - Must be infused on an infusion pump
  - Loading dose should be given in a small volume, and
    continuous infusion should be given in a larger volume

Amiodarone (Cordarone)

- **Common Adult Dose:** 150 mg over 10 minutes, followed by
  360 mg over next 6 hours, followed by 540 mg over next 18
  hours
  - Continue an infusion at 0.5 mg/min until oral preparation
    initiated
- **ACLS Guideline (pulseless V-fib/V-tach):** 300 mg IV push,
  followed by 150 mg IV push after 3–5 minutes
- **Reconstitution:** N/A
- **Solution Amount:** *Loading Dose:* Add 3 ml (150 mg) to 100 ml
  of D_5W for a concentration of 1.5 mg/ml
  Loading Infusion: Add 18 ml (900 mg) to 500 ml of D_5W for
  a concentration of 1.8 mg/ml
- **Compatible Solutions:** D_5W
- **IV Push:** Yes: only in cardiac arrest situation

- **Infusion Time:** *Loading Dose:* Rapidly over 10 minutes; *Loading Infusion:* 360 mg over 6 hours at 1 mg/min, followed by 540 mg over the remaining 18 hours at 0.5 mg/min
- **IVPB:** No—infuse over 24 hours, then maintenance infusion
- **Special Considerations:**
  - Must be administered by volumetric pump
  - Must be administered through an in-line filter
  - Patient must be on cardiac monitoring
  - Do not confuse with **Amrinone**, now called **Inamrinone**

Amphotericin B Cholesteryl Sulfate (Amphotec)

- **Common Adult and Child Dose:** 3–4 mg/kg/day
- **Reconstitution:** Reconstitute 50 mg vials with 10 ml of sterile water for injection and 100 mg vials with 20 ml of sterile water for injection for a final concentration of 5 mg/ml
- **Compatible Solutions:** Further reconstitute with D_5W to a concentration of 0.6 mg/ml
- **IV Push:** No
- **IVPB:** Yes
- **Infusion Time:** 1 mg/kg/hr via infusion pump
- **Special Considerations:**
  - Use a 20 gauge needle, and change for every step of reconstitution
  - Wear gloves while handling
  - Administration through central line is preferable; if a peripheral line must be used, change site for each dose

Amphotericin B Deoxycholate (Fungizone)

- **Common Adult Dose:** 0.25 mg/kg–1.5 mg/kg/day after a test dose of 1 mg
- **Common Child Dose:** 0.25 mg/kg–1 mg/kg/day after a test dose of 0.25 mg
- **Reconstitution:** Reconstitute 50 mg vials with 10 ml of sterile water for injection without bacteriostatic agent for a final concentration of 5 mg/ml

- **Solution Amount:** Further dilute to a concentration of 1 mg per 10 ml of D_5W
- **Compatible Solutions:** D_5W
- **IV Push:** No
- **IVPB:** Yes
- **IV Infusion Time:** 2–6 hours
- **Special Considerations:**
  - Use a 20 gauge needle, and change for every step of reconstitution
  - Wear gloves while handling
  - Administration through central line is preferable; if a peripheral line must be used, change site for each dose
  - If an in-line filter is used, use a 1 micron filter
  - Administer only to hospitalized patients and monitor closely

Amphotericin B Lipid Complex (Abelcet)

- **Common Adult and Child Dose:** 5 mg/kg/day
- **Reconstitution:** Not specified
- **Solution Amount:** Further dilute to a concentration of 1 mg per 10 ml of D_5W
- **Compatible Solutions:** D_5W
- **IV Push:** No
- **IVPB:** Yes
- **IV Infusion Time:** 2.5 mg/kg/hr via infusion pump. If infusion is longer than 2 hours, shake infusion bag every 2 hours to remix
- **Special Considerations:**
  - Withdraw medication from vials with an 18 gauge needle
  - Replace 18 gauge needle with a 5 micron filter needle, and use this needle to inject medication into the IV bag; use filter needle for no more than four vials of medication
  - Does not use an in-line filter
  - Flush IV lines with D_5W before administration, or use separate line

Amphotericin B Liposome (AmBisome)

- **Common Adult and Child Dose:** 3–5 mg/kg/day
- **Reconstitution:** Add 12 ml of sterile water without bacteriostatic agent into a 50 mg vial for a final concentration of 4 mg/ml; immediately shake vial vigorously for at least 30 seconds
- **Compatible Solutions:** Further reconstitute with D_5W to a concentration of 1–2 mg/ml
- **IV Push:** No
- **IVPB:** Yes
- **Infusion Time:** 2 hours; may increase time to 1 hour if patient tolerates administration
- **Special Considerations:**
  - Withdraw solution from vial using a 5 micron filter needle
  - Must be used within 6 hours of dilution
  - Flush existing line with D_5W before administration, or use a separate line

Ampicillin (Omnipen)

- **Common Adult and Child Dose ≥40 kg:** 250–500 mg every 6 hours
- **Common Child dose ≤40 kg:** 25–50 mg/kg/day, divided doses every 6–8 hours
- **Reconstitution:** Add 5 ml of sterile water for injection to each 125, 250, or 500 mg vials or at least 7.4–10 ml of diluent to each 1–2 g vial
- **Solution Amount:** Dilute in at least 50 ml of fluid
- **Compatible Solutions:** D_5W, NaCl, D5/0.45% NaCl, or LR
- **IV Push:** Yes
- **IV Push Rate:** 125–500 ml may be pushed over 3–5 minutes within 1 hour of reconstitution
- **IVPB:** Yes
- **IV Infusion Time:** 10–15 minutes; administer with 4 hours
- **Special Considerations:**
  - Solution is more stable if mixed with NaCl

Ampicillin/Sulbactam (Unasyn)

- **Common Adult and Child Dose ≥ 40 kg:** 1.5 g (1 g ampicillin and 0.5 g sulbactam)–3 g (2 g ampicillin and 1 g sulbactam) every 6 hours for a maximum of 4 g/day
- **Common Child Dose ≤ 1 year old:** 75 mg (50 mg ampicillin and 25 mg sulbactam) per kg every 6 hours
- **Reconstitution:** Add 3.2 ml of sterile water for injection of each 1.5 g vial and 6.4 ml to each 3 g vial for a final concentration of 250 mg ampicillin and 125 mg sulbactam per ml
- **Solution Amount:** 50–100 ml
- **Compatible Solutions:** Dilute immediately for infusion with 0.9% NaCl, D5W, D5/0.45% NaCl, or LR
- **IV Push:** Yes
- **IV Push Rate:** 10–15 minutes
- **IVPB:** Yes
- **Infusion Time:** 15–30 minutes
- **Special Considerations:**
  - Foaming will dissipate upon standing
  - Administer within 1 hour of preparation
  - Rapid administration may cause seizures

Anistreplase (Streptokinase activator complex, Eminase)

- **Common Adult Dose:** 30 U
- **Reconstitution:** Add 5 ml of sterile water—inject to side of vial and swirl gently; do not shake
- **Solution Amount:** No further dilution
- **Compatible Solutions:** Not specified
- **IV Push:** Yes
- **IV Push Rate:** 2–5 minutes directly into vein or into IV line
- **IVPB:** No
- **Special Considerations:** Give within 30 minutes of preparation; cannot be admixed with other medications
  - Must be on a cardiac monitor

Argatroban (Argatroban)

- **Common Adult Dose:** 2 mcg/kg/min as continuous infusion, adjusted based on activated partial thromboplastin time (aPTT); for patients undergoing percutaneous coronary intervention (PCI) give 350 mcg/kg bolus, followed by an infusion of 25 mcg/kg/min
- **Solution Amount:** Each 2.5 ml vial must be diluted in 250 ml; final concentration of infused solution must be 1 mg/1 ml
- **Compatible Solutions:** Dilute immediately for infusion with 0.9% NaCl, D₅W, or LR
- **IV Push:** Yes
- **IV Push Rate:** 3–5 minutes
- **IVPB:** Yes
- **Infusion Time:** 2 mcg/kg/min; 25 mcg/kg/min for PCI patients
- **Special Considerations:**
  - Do not mix with any other medications
  - Protect from light

Atenolol (Tenormin)

- **Common Adult Dose:** 5 mg followed by another 5 mg in 10 minutes
- **Compatible Solutions:** D₅W, 0.9% NaCl, D5/0.9% NaCl; may be diluted for IV push administration is desired
- **IV Push:** Yes
- **IV Push Rate:** 5 mg over 5 minutes
- **Special Considerations:**
  - Diluted solution is stable for 48 hours

Atropine (Atropen)

- **Common Adult and Child ≥20 kg Dose:** *Preanesthesia:* 0.2–1 mg; *Bradycardia:* 0.4–1 mg to a maximum of 3 mg; *Reversal:* 0.6–1.2 mg; *Poisoning:* 1–2 mg to a maximum of 2–6 mg every 5–60 minutes

- **Common Child Dose:** *Bradycardia:* 0.01 mg–0.03 mg/kg for a maximum of 1 mg; *Poisoning:* 0.05 mg/kg every 10–30 minutes as needed
- **IV Push:** Yes
- **IV Push Rate:** 0.6 mg over 1 minute
- **IVPB:** No
- **Special Considerations:**
  - May dilute in 10 ml of sterile water for IV push administration
  - Do not add to IV solution for infusion
  - If given over a longer period than 1 minute, may cause paradoxical bradycardia, which will resolve in 2 minutes

Azathioprine (Imuran)

- **Common Adult and Child Dose:** Initially 3–5 mg/kg/day; maintenance dose 1–3 mg/kg/day
- **Reconstitution:** Reconstitute 100 mg with 10 ml of sterile water for injection
- **Solution Amount:** 50 ml
- **Compatible Solutions:** D₅W, 0.9% NaCl, 0.45% NaCl
- **IV Push:** No
- **IVPB:** Yes
- **IVPB Infusion Time:** 30–60 minutes
- **Special Considerations:**
  - Solution must be prepared in a biological cabinet wearing gloves, gown, and mask at all times when handling solution
  - Discard equipment in specially designated containers
  - Swirl vial gently until completely dissolved
  - Do not confuse with Imdur

Azithromycin (Zithromax)

- **Common Adult Dose:** 500 mg every 24 hours for 1-2 days
- **Reconstitution:** Add 4.8 ml of sterile water for injection to the 500 mg vial and shake until dissolved; the final concentration will be 100 mg/ml

- **Solution Amount:** 250 ml or 500 ml for a final concentration of 2 mg/ml or 1 mg/ml
- **Compatible Solutions:** 0.9% NaCl, 0.45% NaCl, D₅W, LR, D5/0.45% NaCl, D5/LR
- **IV Push:** No
- **IVPB:** Yes
- **IVPB Infusion Time:** 1 mg/ml solution over 3 hours or the 2 mg/ml solution over 1 hour
- **Special Considerations:**
  - Do not administer solutions containing particulate matter
  - Solution is stable for 24 hours at room temperature and 7 days if refrigerated

Basiliximab (Simulect)

- **Common Adult and Child (≥35 kg) Dose:** 20 mg 2 hours before transplantation, repeated 4 days after transplantation
- **Common Child Dose (<35 kg):** 10 mg 2 hours before transplantation, repeated 4 days after transplantation
- **Reconstitution:** Add 2.5 ml of sterile water to the 10 mg vial and 5 ml of sterile water to the 20 mg vial; shake gently to dissolve
- **Solution Amount:** 25 or 50 ml
- **Compatible Solutions:** D₅W or 0.9% NaCl
- **IV Push:** Yes: may be administered without further dilution
- **IV Push Rate:** Not specified but may be associated with nausea, vomiting, and IV site pain
- **IVPB:** Yes
- **IV Infusion Time:** 20–30 minutes
- **Special Considerations:**
  - Do not shake bag after mixing
  - Administer within 4 hours
  - Typically administered concurrently with cyclosporine and corticosteroids

Benztropine (Cogentin)

- **Common Adult Dose:** 1–2 mg
- **Common Child Dose:** N/A
- **IV Push:** Yes
- **IV Push Rate:** 1 mg over 1 minute
- **IVPB:** No
- **Special Considerations:**
  - IV rate is rarely used because the IM route onset is the same as the IV onset

Betamethasone (Celestone)

- **Common Adult Dose:** Up to 9 mg
- **Common Child Dose:** N/A
- **Reconstitution:** May be administered undiluted
- **Solution Amount:** Not specified
- **Compatible Solutions:** D$_5$W, 0.9% NaCl, Ringer's solution, D5/Ringer's solution, D5/LR
- **IV Push:** Yes
- **IVPB:** Yes
- **IV Push Rate:** Over at least 1 minute
- **IV Infusion Time:** Not specified
- **Special Considerations:** Only betamethasone phosphate may be given intravenously

Biperiden (Akineton)

- **Common Adult Dose:** 2 mg may be repeated every 3 minutes up to a total of 4 doses in 24 hours
- **IV Push:** Yes: may be administered without further dilution
- **IV Push Rate:** Administer each dose over at least 1 minute to prevent hypotension and mild bradycardia
- **IVPB:** No

Bivalirudin (Angiomax)

- **Common Adult Dose:** 1 mg/kg as a bolus injection, followed by a 4 hour infusion at 2.5 mg/kg/hr; this may be followed by a second infusion at 2 mg/kg/hr for 20 hours
- **Reconstitution:** Add 5 ml of sterile water for injection to each vial of 250 mg; swirl until dissolved
- **Solution Amount:** 500 ml
- **Compatible Solutions:** D_5W, 0.9% NaCl
- **IV Push:** Yes
- **IV Push Rate:** Not specified—administer as a bolus dose
- **IVPB:** Yes
- **IV Infusion Time:** First infusion over 4 hours; if ordered, a second infusion will be infused over 20 hours
- **Special Considerations:**
  - Use a separate line for administration—do not mix with other medications

Botulism Immune Globulin (BabyBIG)

- **Common Child Dose:** <1 yr: 1 ml/kg as a single infusion
- **Reconstitution:** Add 2 ml of sterile water to lyophilized powder—50 mg/ml—by using a double-ended transfer device or large syringe; add sterile water to side of vial; rotate vial gently to wet the powder—do not shake
- **Solution Amount:** Not specified
- **Compatible Solutions:** Not specified
- **IV Push:** Yes
- **IV Push Rate:** Use filter (18 micron) to administer; begin slowly at 0.5 ml/kg/hr or 25 mg/kg/hr—undesirable reactions within 15 minutes; rate may be increased to 1.0 ml/kg/hr or 50 mg/kg/hr; infusion should take a total of 67.5 minutes
- **IVPB:** No
- **Special Considerations:** Infusion should begin within 2 hours of reconstitution and complete within 4 hours; closely monitor patient after each rate change

Bumetanide (Bumex)

- **Common Adult Dose:** 0.5–1 mg/day up to 10 mg/day
- **Reconstitution:** N/A
- **Solution Amount:** Not specified
- **Compatible Solutions:** D₅W, 0.9% NaCl, LR
- **IV Push:** Yes; may be administered undiluted
- **IV Push Rate:** Slowly over 2 minutes
- **IVPB:** Yes
- **IV Infusion Time:** May be administered over 12 hours for patients with renal impairment; otherwise, rate unspecified
- **Special Considerations:**
  - Do not confuse with buprenorphine (Buprenex)

Buprenorphine (Buprenex)

- **Common Adult Dose:** 0.3 mg every 4–6 hours as needed
- **Common Pediatric Dose:** 2–6 mcg every 4–6 hours as needed
- **Compatible Solutions:** D₅W, 0.9% NaCl, D5/0.9% NaCl, LR, Ringer's injection
- **IV Push:** Yes
- **IV Push Rate:** Not specified—administer slowly
- **IVPB:** No
- **Special Considerations:**
  - May be administered undiluted
  - Rapid administration may cause respiratory depression, hypotension, and cardiac arrest

Butorphanol (Stadol)

- **Common Adult Dose:** 1 mg every 3–4 hours as needed
- **Reconstitution:** N/A
- **Solution Amount:** Not specified
- **Compatible Solutions:** Not specified
- **IV Push:** Yes; may be administered undiluted
- **IV Push Rate:** Over 3–5 minutes

- **IVPB:** No
- **Special Considerations:**
  - May be administered undiluted
  - Rapid administration may cause respiratory depression, hypotension, and cardiac arrest

Ca-DTPA (Pentetate Calcium Trisodium)

- **Common Adult Dose (12 years and older):** Length of treatment depends on extent and response of contamination; give 1 g dose followed by Zn-DTPA; if Zn-DTPA not available, continue with 1 g Ca-DTPA daily
- **Common Child Dose <12 years:** Length of treatment depends on extent and response of contamination; 14 mg/kg single dose and not to surpass 1 g dose followed by Zn-DTPA; if Zn-DTPA not available, continue Ca-DTPA 14 mg/kg daily
- **Reconstitution:** Not specified
- **Solution Amount:** 100–250 ml of a compatible solution
- **Compatible Solutions:** D_5W, LR, 0.9% NaCl
- **IV Push:** Yes
- **IV Push Rate:** Give over 3–4 minutes
- **IVPB:** Yes
- **IV Infusion Time:** Slow infusion
- **Special Considerations:** If more than one dose must be given, supplements of zinc must be given concurrently; give mineral or vitamin supplements as needed; patient should drink plenty of fluids and void frequently to dilute urine and prevent radiation damage to bladder; instruct patient to flush toilet several times after use

Calcium Chloride

- **Common Adult Dose:** *Hypocalcemia:* 7–14 mEq; *Hypocalcemic Tetany:* 4.5–16 mEq; *Hyperkalemia with Cardiac Toxicity:* 2.25–14 mEq; *Hypermagnesemia:* 7 mEq
- **Common Pediatric Dose:** *Hypocalcemia:* 1–7 mEq; *Hypocalcemic Tetany:* 0.5–0.7 mEq 3–4 times/day

- **Compatible Solutions:** D₅W, 0.9% NaCl, D5/0.45% NaCl, LR, D₁₀W, D5/0.2% NaCl, D5/0.9% NaCl, D5/LR
- **IV Push:** Yes
- **IV Push Rate:** 0.7–1.4 mEq/min
- **IV Push Rate for children:** 0.5 ml/min
- **IVPB:** No
- **Special Considerations:**
■ Give through a small-bore needle into a large vein to minimize phlebitis—do not administer through a scalp vein
■ Warm to body temperature
■ May cause site burning, peripheral vasodilation, drop in blood pressure (BP)
■ Patients should remain recumbent for 30–60 minutes after IV administration
■ Rapid administration can result in cardiac arrest

Calcium Gluceptate

- **Common Adult Dose:** Hypocalcemia: 7–14 mEq; Hypocalcemic Tetany: 4.5–16 mEq; Hyperkalemia with Cardiac Toxicity: 2.25–14 mEq; Hypermagnesemia: 7 mEq
- **Common Pediatric Dose:** Hypocalcemia: 1–7 mEq; Hypocalcemic Tetany: 0.5–0.7 mEq 3–4 times per day
- **Compatible Solutions:** D₅W, 0.9% NaCl, D5/0.9% NaCl, LR, D₁₀W, D5/0.2% NaCl, D5/0.45% NaCl, D5/LR
- **IVPB:** Yes
- **IV Push:** may be administered undiluted
- **IV Push Rate:** 2 ml/min (1.8 mEq/min)
- **IV Push Rate for Children:** 0.5 ml/min (0.45 mEq/min)
- **IVPB Rate:** Not to exceed 200 mg/min
- **Special Considerations:**
■ Warm to body temperature
■ Give through a small-bore needle into a large vein to minimize phlebitis—do not administer through a scalp vein
■ May cause site burning, peripheral vasodilation, drop in BP
■ Patients should remain recumbent for 30–60 minutes after IV administration
■ Rapid administration can result in cardiac arrest

Calcium Gluconate (Kalcinate)

- **Common Adult Dose:** *Hypocalcemia:* 7–14 mEq; *Hypocalcemic Tetany:* 4.5–16 mEq; *Hyperkalemia with Cardiac Toxicity:* 2.25–14 mEq; *Hypermagnesemia:* 7 mEq
- **Common Pediatric Dose:** *Hypocalcemia:* 1–7 MEq; *Hypocalcemic Tetany:* 0.5–0.7 mEq 3–4 times per day
- **Solution Amount:** 1000 ml
- **Compatible Solutions:** D$_5$W, 0.9% NaCl, D5/0.9% NaCl, LR, D$_{10}$W, D$_{20}$W, D5/LR
- **IV Push:** Yes
- **IV Push Rate:** Do not exceed 1.5–2 ml/min
- **IVPB:** Yes
- **IVPB Rate:** Do not exceed rate 200 mg/min over 12–24 hours
- **Special Considerations:** Same as calcium gluceptate

Caspofungin (Cancidas)

- **Common Adult Dose:** 70 mg initially, followed by 50 mg daily
- **Common Child Dose:** N/A
- **Reconstitution:** Add 10.5 ml of 0.9% NaCl or bacteriostatic water to the 70 mg or 50 mg vial
- **Solution Amount:** 250 ml or 100 ml if medically necessary
- **Compatible Solutions:** 0.225% NaCl, 0.45% NaCl, 0.9% NaCl, LR
- **IV Push:** No
- **IVPB:** Yes
- **IV Infusion Time:** 1 hour
- **Special Considerations:** white cake should dissolve completely when reconstituting
  - Mix gently until solution is clear
  - Refrigerated solutions must be used within 24 hours
  - Room temperature solutions must be used within 1 hour

Cefazolin (Ancef)

- **Common Adult Dose:** 250 mg–1.5 g every 6–8 hours
- **Common Child Dose:** 6.25 mg–25 mg/kg every 6 hours or 8.3 mg–33.3 mg/kg every 8 hours
- **Reconstitution:** Not specified
- **Solution Amount:** 50–100 ml
- **Compatible Solutions:** D5W, D5/0.45% NaCl, D5/0.9% NaCl, D10W, D5/0.25% NaCl, 0.9% NaCl, LR, D5/LR
- **IV Push:** No
- **IVPB:** Yes
- **IV Infusion Time:** 30–60 minutes
- **Special Considerations:** N/A

Cefepime (Maxipime)

- **Common Adult Dose:** 0.5 mg–1 g every 12 hours
- **Common Child Dose:** 50 mg/kg every 8–12 hours
- **Reconstitution:** Not specified
- **Solution Amount:** 50–100 ml
- **Compatible Solutions:** D5W, D5/0.9% NaCl, 0.9% NaCl, D5/LR, D5/Normosol R or D5/Normosol M, M/6 Sodium lactate injection
- **IV Push:** No
- **IVPB:** Yes
- **IV Infusion Time:** 30 minutes
- **Special Considerations:** Stable for 24 hours at room temperature and 7 days if refrigerated

Cefmetazole (Zefazone)

- **Common Adult Dose:** 2 g every 6–12 hours
- **Common Child Dose:** N/A
- **Reconstitution:** Not specified
- **Solution Amount:** 50–100 ml
- **Compatible Solutions:** D5W, 0.9% NaCl, LR

- **IV Push:** No
- **IVPB:** Yes
- **IV Infusion Time:** 10–60 minutes
- **Special Considerations:** Stable for 24 hours at room temperature

Cefonicid (Monocid)

- **Common Adult Dose:** 0.5–2 g every 24 hours
- **Common Child Dose:** N/A
- **Reconstitution:** Not specified
- **Solution Amount:** 50–100 ml
- **Compatible Solutions:** D_5W, $D_{10}W$, D5/0.25% NaCl, D5/0.45% NaCl, D5/0.9% NaCl, 0.9% NaCl, LR, D5/LR
- **IV Push:** No
- **IVPB:** Yes
- **IV Infusion Time:** 20–30 minutes
- **Special Considerations:** Reconstituted solution may be colorless to slightly amber
  - Solution is stable at room temperature for 24 hours and 72 hours if refrigerated

Cefoperazone (Cefobid)

- **Common Adult Dose:** 1–6 g every 12 hours
- **Common Child Dose:** N/A
- **Reconstitution:** Reconstitute each gram with at least 2.8 ml of sterile bacteriostatic water or saline or 0.9% NaCl; shake vigorously and allow to stand until visually clear
- **Solution Amount:** Further dilute in 20–40 ml
- **Compatible Solutions:** D_5W, $D_{10}W$, D5/0.25% NaCl, D5/0.9% NaCl, 0.9% NaCl, LR, D5/LR
- **IV Push:** No
- **IVPB:** Yes
- **IV Infusion Time:** 15–30 minutes
- **Special Considerations:** For continuous infusion solutions, should have a concentration of 2–25 mg/ml

MED

Cefotaxime (Claforan)

- **Common Adult Dose:** 1–2 g every 4, 6, or 8 hours
- **Common Child Dose:** 8.3–45 mg/kg every 4–6 hours
- **Reconstitution:** Not specified
- **Solution Amount:** 50–100 ml
- **Compatible Solutions:** D_5W, $D_{10}W$, D5/0.25% NaCl, D5/0.9% NaCl, 0.9% NaCl, D5/0.45% NaCl, LR
- **IV Push:** No
- **IVPB:** Yes
- **IV Infusion Time:** 20–30 minutes
- **Special Considerations:** Solution may appear light yellow to amber
  - Solution stable for 24 hours at room temperature and 5 days if refrigerated

Cefotetan (Cefotan)

- **Common Adult Dose:** 500 mg–3 g every 12–24 hours
- **Common Child Dose:** N/A
- **Reconstitution:** Not specified
- **Solution Amount:** 50–100 ml
- **Compatible Solutions:** D_5W, 0.9% NaCl
- **IV Push:** No
- **IVPB:** Yes
- **IV Infusion Time:** 20–30 minutes
- **Special Considerations:** Reconstituted solution may be yellow
  - Solution is stable for 24 hours at room temperature and 96 hours if refrigerated

Cefoxitin (Mefoxin)

- **Common Adult Dose:** 1–3 g every 4, 6, or 8 hours
- **Common Child Dose:** 13.3–26.7 mg/kg every 4 hours or 20–40 mg/kg every 6 hours
- **Reconstitution:** Not specified
- **Solution Amount:** 50–100 ml
- **Compatible Solutions:** D_5W, $D_{10}W$, D5/0.25% NaCl, D5/0.45% NaCl, D5/0.9% NaCl, 0.9% NaCl, LR, D5/LR, Ringer's solution
- **IV Push:** No
- **IVPB:** Yes
- **IV Infusion Time:** 15–30 minutes
- **Special Considerations:** May be diluted in 500–1000 ml for continuous infusion
    - Stable at room temperature for 24 hours and 1 week if refrigerated

Ceftazidime (Tazidime)

- **Common Adult Dose:** 500 mg–2 g every 8–12 hours
- **Common Child Dose:** 30–50 mg/kg every 8 hours
- **Reconstitution:** Not specified
- **Solution Amount:** Further dilute to a solution of 1 g/10 ml
- **Compatible Solutions:** D_5W, $D_{10}W$, D5/0.25% NaCl, D5/0.45% NaCl, D5/0.9% NaCl, 0.9% NaCl, LR
- **IV Push:** No
- **IVPB:** Yes
- **IV Infusion Time:** 15–30 minutes
- **Special Considerations:** Dilution causes CO_2 to form inside the vial, resulting in positive pressure in the vial; this may require venting the vial to preserve sterility; solution stable 18 hours at room temperature and 7 days if refrigerated

Ceftizoxime (Cefizox)

- **Common Adult Dose:** 1–4 g every 8–12 hours
- **Common Child Dose:** 50 mg/kg every 6–8 hours (not to exceed 200 mg/day)
- **Reconstitution:** Not specified
- **Solution Amount:** 50–100 ml
- **Compatible Solutions:** D_5W, $D_{10}W$, D5/0.25% NaCl, D5/0.45% NaCl, D5/0.9% NaCl, 0.9% NaCl, LR
- **IV Push:** No
- **IVPB:** Yes
- **IV Infusion Time:** 15–30 minutes
- **Special Considerations:** Solution stable 8 hours at room temperature and 48 hours if refrigerated

Ceftriaxone (Rocephin)

- **Common Adult Dose:** 0.5–2 g every 12–24 hours
- **Common Child Dose:** 25–100 mg/kg every 12 hours
- **Reconstitution:** Reconstitute every 250 mg vial with 2.4 ml; every 500 mg vial with 4.8 ml; each 1 g vial with 9.6 ml; and each 2 g vial with 19.2 ml with 0.9% NaCl, D_5W, or sterile water for injection
- **Solution Amount:** Further dilute in 50–100 ml
- **Compatible Solutions:** D_5W, $D_{10}W$, D5/0.45% NaCl, D5/0.9% NaCl, 0.9% NaCl, LR
- **IV Push:** No
- **IVPB:** Yes
- **IV Infusion Time:** 15–30 minutes for adults and 10–30 minutes for children
- **Special Considerations:** Solution may appear light amber to yellow
- ■ Solution is stable for 3 days at room temperature

Cefuroxime (Ceftin)

- **Common Adult Dose:** 750 mg–3 g every 8 hours
- **Common Child Dose:** 15–80 mg/kg every 8–12 hours
- **Reconstitution:** Not specified
- **Solution Amount:** 100 ml
- **Compatible Solutions:** D₅W, D₁₀W, D5/0.45% NaCl, D5/0.9% NaCl, 0.9% NaCl
- **IV Push:** No
- **IVPB:** Yes
- **IV Infusion Time:** 15–60 minutes
- **Special Considerations:** May be diluted in 500–1000 ml for continuous infusion
  - Stable at room temperature for 24 hours and 1 week if refrigerated

Cephapirin (Velosef)

- **Common Adult Dose:** 0.5 mg–1 g every 4–6 hours
- **Common Child Dose:** 10–20 mg/kg every 6 hours
- **Reconstitution:** Not specified
- **Solution Amount:** 50–100 ml
- **Compatible Solutions:** D₅W, D₁₀W, D5/0.25% NaCl, D5/0.45% NaCl, D5/0.9% NaCl, 0.9% NaCl, D5/LR
- **IV Push:** No
- **IVPB:** Yes
- **IV Infusion Time:** 15–20 minutes
- **Special Considerations:** Can be diluted in 500–1000 ml for continuous infusion

Chlordiazepoxide (Librium)

- **Common Adult Dose:** 25–100 mg initially and then may be repeated in 2–4 hours
- **Common Child Dose:** 25–50 mg per dose
- **Reconstitution:** Reconstitute 100 mg in 5 ml of 0.9% NaCl or sterile water for injection
- **Solution Amount:** N/A

- **Compatible Solutions**: Not specified
- **IV Push**: Yes
- **IVP Rate**: Push slowly over at least 1 minute
- **IVPB**: No
- **Special Considerations**: Do not use the IM diluent for IV administration
  - Use parenteral solution immediately after reconstitution, and discard unused portion

Chlorpheniramine (Chlor-Trimeton)

- **Common Adult Dose**: 5–40 mg as a single dose; do not exceed 40 mg/day
- **Common Child Dose**: N/A
- **Reconstitution**: May be given undiluted
- **Solution Amount**: N/A
- **Compatible Solutions**: Not specified
- **IV Push**: Yes
- **IVPB**: No
- **IVP Rate**: Administer each 10 mg dose over 1 minute
- **Special Considerations**: Use only the 10 mg dose for IV administration

Cidofovir (Vistide)

- **Common Adult Dose**: 5 mg/kg once a week for 2 weeks followed by 5 mg/kg every 2 weeks
- **Common Child Dose**: N/A
- **Reconstitution**: N/A
- **Solution Amount**: 100 ml
- **Compatible Solutions**: 0.9% NaCl
- **IV Push**: No
- **IVPB**: Yes
- **IV Infusion Time**: 1 hour
- **Special Considerations**: Must be given with probenicid
  - Solution is stable for 24 hours if refrigerated
  - Allow solution to come to room temperature before administration

Cimetidine (Tagamet)

- **Common Adult Dose:** 300–600 mg q 6 hours up to 12 g/day; may be given as a continuous infusion of 900 mg over 24 hours, preceded by a 150 mg bolus
- **Common Child Dose:** 5–10 mg/kg q 6–8 hours
- **Reconstitution:** N/A
- **Solution Amount:** 50 ml; continuous infusion: 100–1000 ml
- **Compatible Solutions:** D_5W, $D_{10}W$, D5/0.25% NaCl, D5/0.45% NaCl, D5/0.9% NaCl, 0.9% NaCl, LR, D5/LR, sodium bicarbonate
- **IV Push:** Yes: diluted in 20 ml of 0.9% NaCl for injection
- **IV Push Rate:** Administer over at least 5 minutes
- **IVPB:** Yes
- **IV Infusion Time:** 15–20 minutes
- **Special Considerations:** Do not administer solution that is discolored or that contains precipitate

Ciprofloxacin (Cipro)

- **Common Adult Dose:** 200–400 mg q 12 hours
- **Common Child Dose:** 10 mg/kg every 12 hours
- **Reconstitution:** Dilute to a concentration of 1–2 mg/ml
- **Solution Amount:** Dilute to a concentration of 1–2 mg/ml
- **Compatible Solutions:** 0.9% NaCl
- **IV Push:** No
- **IVPB:** Yes
- **IV Infusion Time:** 60 minutes
- **Special Considerations:** Administer into a large vein

Clindamycin (Cleocin)

- **Common Adult Dose:** 300–900 mg every 8 hours; P. carinii *Pneumonia*: 2400–2700 mg/day in divided dose; *Toxoplasmosis* 1200–4800 mg/day in divided doses
- **Common Child Dose:** 3.75–13.3 mg/kg every 6–8 hours
- **Reconstitution:** N/A
- **Solution Amount:** 300–600 mg dilute in at least 50 ml; 900–1200 mg dilute in at least 100 ml
- **Compatible Solutions:** D5W, D10W, D5/0.45% NaCl, D5/0.9% NaCl, 0.9% NaCl, LR, D5/Ringer's solution
- **IV Push:** No
- **IVPB:** Yes
- **IV Infusion Time:** Each 300 mg should be infused over at least 10 minutes; may be administered as a continuous infusion 0.75–1.25 mg/min
- **Special Considerations:** Crystals may occur if solution is refrigerated; do not administer with crystals in solution—warm to room temperature, then administer

Colchicine

- **Common Adult Dose:** 2 mg initially, followed by 0.5–1 mg every 6–12 hours
- **Common Child Dose:** N/A
- **Reconstitution:** May be administered undiluted, but if a lower concentration is desired, dilute to a volume of 10–20 ml with 0.9% NaCl
- **Solution Amount:** N/A
- **Compatible Solutions:** N/A
- **IV Push:** Yes
- **IV Rate:** Slowly over 2–10 minutes
- **IVPB:** No
- **Special Considerations:** Do not administer oral and IV colchicine concurrently
■ Avoid extravasation—may cause necrosis of soft tissue

Cyclosporine (Sandimmune)

- **Common Adult and Child Dose:** 2–6 mg/kg/day initially; change to po as soon as possible
- **Reconstitution:** Dilute each 1 ml of concentrate immediately before use with 20–100 ml of D$_5$W or 0.9% NaCl for injection
- **Solution Amount:** Not specified
- **Compatible Solutions:** D$_5$W, 0.9% NaCl
- **IV Push:** No
- **IVPB:** Yes
- **IV Infusion Time:** Infuse slowly over 2–6 hours via infusion pump; may be administered over 24 hours
- **Special Considerations:** Solution stable 6 hours in a polyvinylchloride container for 12 hours and in a glass container at room temperature

Daclizumab (Zenapax)

- **Common Adult and Child Dose:** 1 mg/kg with first dose given no more than 24 hours before transplantation, then every 2 weeks for a total of 5 doses
- **Reconstitution:** Dilute with 50 ml or 0.9% NaCl; gently invert bag to mix; do not shake to avoid foaming
- **Solution Amount:** 50 ml
- **Compatible Solutions:** 0.9% NaCl
- **IV Push:** No
- **IVPB:** Yes
- **IV Infusion Time:** 15 minutes
- **Special Considerations:** Solution is clear and colorless; do not administer if not clear and colorless
  - Administer within 4 hours
  - May be refrigerated for up to 24 hours
  - Discard after 24 hours
  - If administered in a nondedicated line, flush with 0.9% NaCl before and after administration

Dantrolene (Dantrium)

- **Common Adult and Child Dose:** 1–3 mg/kg; not to exceed 10 mg/kg
- **Reconstitution:** Reconstitute each 20 mg with 60 ml of sterile water for injection without bacteriostatic agent for a final concentration of 333 mcg/ml
- **Solution Amount:** 60 ml
- **Compatible Solutions:** Not specified
- **IV Push:** Yes
- **IV Push Rate:** Rapid IV push through Y tubing or a three-way stopcock
- **IVPB:** Yes
- **IV Infusion Time:** Intermittent infusion is used prophylactically before anesthesia—administer over 1 hour before anesthesia
- **Special Considerations:** Shake until solution is clear
- Medication is very irritating to tissue; monitor carefully for extravasation
- Solution must be used within 6 hours
- Protect solution from direct light

Daptomycin (Cubicin)

- **Common Adult Dose:** 4 mg/kg q 24 hours
- **Reconstitution:** Add 5 ml 0.9% NaCl to 250 mg vial, and 10 ml 0.9% NaCl to 500 mg vial
- **Solution Amount:** 50–100 ml of a compatible solution
- **Compatible Solutions:** 0.9% NaCl, LR
- **IV Push:** No
- **IVPB:** Yes
- **IV Infusion Time:** 30 minutes
- **Special Considerations:** Incompatible with dextrose solutions; do not administer if solution is cloudy or if precipitate is present

Darbepoetin (Aranesp)

- **Common Adult Dose:** 0.45 mcg/kg every week—adjust dose to target hemoglobin
- **Common Child Dose:** N/A
- **Reconstitution:** Administer undiluted
- **Solution Amount:** N/A
- **Compatible Solutions:** Not specified
- **IV Push:** Yes
- **IV Push Rate:** Not specified
- **IVPB:** Yes
- **IV Infusion Time:** Not specified
- **Special Considerations:** Do not administer in conjunction with other drugs or solutions

Desmopressin (DDAVP)

- **Common Adult and Child Dose:** *Primary Enuresis:* 2–4 μg/day in 2 divided doses; *Antihemorrhagic:* 0.3 mcg/kg—repeated as necessary
- **Reconstitution:** N/A
- **Solution Amount:** 50 ml for adults and 10 ml for children under 10 kg
- **Compatible Solutions:** 0.9% NaCl
- **IV Push:** Yes
- **IVPB:** Yes
- **IV Push Rate:** Over 1 minute
- **IV Infusion Time:** 15–30 minutes
- **Special Considerations:** Desmopressin has 10 times the antidiuretic effect of intranasal desmopressin

Dexamethasone (Decadron)

- **Common Adult Dose:** 10 mg as an initial dose, followed by 4 mg every 6 hours, decreasing to 2 mg every 8–12 hours, then changing to an oral dose

- **Common Child Dose:** N/A
- **Reconstitution:** May be given undiluted
- **Solution Amount:** Not specified
- **Compatible Solutions:** D_5W, 0.9% NaCl
- **IV Push:** Yes
- **IV Push Rate:** Over 1 minute
- **IVPB:** Yes
- **IV Infusion Time:** Not specified
- **Special Considerations:** Do not administer suspension IV (dexamethasone acetate)
  - Diluted solutions should be given within 24 hours

Dexmedetomidine (Precedex)

- **Common Adult Dose:** Loading dose—1 mcg/kg over 10 minutes, followed by an infusion of 0.2–0.7 mcg/kg/hr
- **Common Child Dose:** N/A
- **Reconstitution:** To prepare solution, withdraw 2 ml of the medication and add to 48 ml of 0.9% NaCl, for a total of 50 ml
- **Solution Amount:** 48 ml
- **Compatible Solutions:** 0.9% NaCl
- **IV Push:** No
- **IVPB:** Yes
- **IV Infusion Time:** Loading dose—over 10 minutes; maintenance 0.2–0.7 mcg/kg/hr to achieve desired sedation
- **Special Considerations:** Should be administered only in an intensive care setting with continuous monitoring
  - Administer via infusion pump

Diazepam (Valium)

- **Common Adult Dose:** 2.5–20 mg repeated every 10–15 minutes until desired effect, for a maximum dose of 30 mg; may repeat regimen in 2–4 hours
- **Common Child Dose:** 0.2–1 mg every 5 minutes to a maximum of 5–10 mg; may repeat in 2–4 hours

- **Reconstitution:** Administer undiluted
- **Solution Amount:** N/A
- **Compatible Solutions:** N/A
- **IV Push:** Yes
- **IV Push Rate:** Adults—5 mg/min; Children—total dose over 3–5 minutes
- **IVPB:** Not recommended due to precipitation in IV fluids and absorption of diazepam by tubing and infusion bags
- **Special Considerations:** Resuscitation equipment should be available when giving diazepam intravenously
  - Sterile emulsion for injection (Dizac) for IV use only
  - Do not dilute
  - Do not use filter to infuse
  - Administer within 6 hours of drawing up medication
  - Flush line at end of infusion to clear medication

Digoxin (Lanoxin)

- **Common Adult Dose:** 0.6–1 mg; loading dose should be given as 50% of the dose initially and then fractions given every 4–8 hours until desired dose achieved
- **Common Child Dose:** 15–35 mcg/kg; loading dose should be given as 50% of the dose initially and then fractions given every 4–8 hours until desired dose achieved
- **Reconstitution:** May be given undiluted, or each 1 ml may be diluted with 4 ml of fluid
- **Solution Amount:** N/A
- **Compatible Solutions:** Sterile water, D_5W, 0.9% NaCl, LR
- **IV Push:** Yes
- **IV Push Rate:** Each dose should be administered over 5 minutes
- **IVPB:** No
- **Special Considerations:** Do not use solution that is discolored or that contains precipitate
  - Do not administer with other drugs

Digoxin Immune Fab (Digibind, DigiFab)

- **Common Adult and Child Dose:** 228 mg (6 vials)—800 mg (20 vials), depending on the type of toxicity being treated
- **Reconstitution:** Reconstitute each vial with 4 ml of sterile water for injection and shake gently
- **Solution Amount:** Not specified; for children, vial may be diluted with 34-36 ml of solution for a concentration of 1 mg/ml
- **Compatible Solutions:** 0.9% NaCl
- **IV Push:** Only if cardiac arrest is imminent!
- **IV Push Rate:** Rapid IV push if cardiac arrest is imminent
- **IVPB:** Yes
- **IV Infusion Time:** 15-30 minutes
- **Special Considerations:** Solution stable 4 hours if refrigerated

Dihydroergotamine (Migranal)

- **Common Adult Dose:** 0.5 mg; may repeat in 1 hour to a total of 3 mg (not to exceed 2 mg/day or 6 mg/week)
- **Common Child Dose:** ≥6 yr: 0.25–0.5 mg 1–2 doses given q 20 minutes
- **Reconstitution:** May be administered undiluted
- **Compatible Solutions:** Not specified
- **IV Push:** Yes
- **IV Push Rate:** Over 1 minute
- **IVPB:** No

Diltiazem (Cardizem)

- **Common Adult Dose:** 0.25 mg/kg; may give a higher dose of 0.33 mg/kg in 15 minutes; may follow with a continuous infusion of 5–15 mg/hr
- **Common Child Dose:** N/A
- **Reconstitution:** May be administered undiluted
- **Solution Amount:** Continuous infusions—125 mg in 100 ml, 250 mg in 250 ml or 500 ml
- **Compatible Solutions:** D5W, D5/0.45% NaCl, 0.9% NaCl

- **IV Push:** Yes
- **IV Push Rate:** Over 2 minutes
- **IVPB:** Yes
- **IV Infusion Time:** Initial infusion should be infused at 10 mg/hr, followed by an infusion rate of 5–15 mg/hr
- **Special Considerations:** Solution stable 24 hours at room temperature or refrigerated

Dimenhydrinate (Dinate)

- **Common Adult Dose:** 50 mg every 4 hours
- **Common Child Dose:** 1.25 mg/kg every 6 hours
- **Reconstitution:** Diluted 50 mg in 10 ml of 0.9% NaCl for injection
- **Solution Amount:** N/A
- **Compatible Solutions:** N/A
- **IV Push:** Yes
- **IV Push Rate:** Inject over 2 minutes
- **IVPB:** No
- **Special Considerations:** May cause drowsiness

Diphenhydramine (Benadryl)

- **Common Adult Dose:** 10–100 mg every 2–3 hours; not to exceed 400 mg/day
- **Common Child Dose:** 1.25 mg/kg 4 times a day; not to exceed 300 mg/day
- **Reconstitution:** May be given undiluted
- **Solution Amount:** Not specified
- **Compatible Solutions:** D_5W, $D_{10}W$, D5/0.25% NaCl, D5/0.45% NaCl, D5/0.9% NaCl, 0.45% NaCl, 0.9% NaCl, LR, Ringer's solution, D5/Ringer's solution
- **IV Push:** Yes
- **IV Push Rate:** 25 mg/min
- **IVPB:** Yes
- **IV Infusion Time:** Not specified
- **Special Considerations:** Do not confuse with **Benylin**

Dipyridamole (Persantine)

- **Common Adult Dose:** 570 mcg/kg; maximum dose—60 mg
- **Reconstitution:** N/A
- **Solution Amount:** Dilute at least a 1:2 ratio for a total volume of 20–50 ml
- **Compatible Solutions:** D5W, 0.9% NaCl
- **IV Push:** No
- **IVPB:** Yes
- **IV Infusion Time:** 4 minutes
- **Special Considerations:** Monitor vital signs and at least one lead of EKG during and 10–15 minutes after infusion
- If severe chest pain occurs, administer IV aminophylline
- If chest pain unrelieved with aminophylline, administer nitroglycerine
- If chest pain still unrelieved, treat as a myocardial infarction

Dobutamine (Dobutrex)

- **Common Adult and Child Dose:** 0.5–40 mcg/kg/min titrated to desired response every few minutes
- **Reconstitution:** Reconstitute a 250 mg vial with 10 ml of sterile water for injection or D5W for injection
- **Solution Amount:** Dilute in at least 50 ml; concentration should not exceed 5 mg/ml
- **Compatible Solutions:** D5W, 0.45% NaCl, D5/0.45% NaCl, D5/0.9% NaCl, 0.9% NaCl, LR, D5/LR, sodium lactate
- **IV Push:** No
- **IVPB:** Yes
- **IV Infusion Time:** Titrate dose to desired effect per dose limitations
- **Special Considerations:** Must be infused via infusion pump
- Administer into a large vein
- Have a second practitioner check infusion pump settings
- Solution may have a slight pink color
- Stable at room temperature for 24 hours

Dopamine (Intropin)

- **Common Adult Dose:** Renal Vasodilation Effect: 0.5–3 mcg/mg/min; Peripheral Vasoconstrictive Effect: 2–10 mcg/kg/min
- **Common Child Dose:** Renal Vasodilation Effect: 0.5–3 mcg/mg/min; Peripheral Vasoconstrictive Effect: 5–20 mcg/kg/min
- **Reconstitution:** N/A
- **Solution Amount:** Dilute 200–400 mg in 250–500 ml with concentrations ranging from 0.08–3.2 mg/ml
- **Compatible Solutions:** D_5W, D5/0.45% NaCl, D5/0.9% NaCl, 0.9% NaCl, LR, D5/LR
- **IV Push:** No
- **IVPB:** Yes: continuous infusion only
- **IV Infusion Time:** Titrate to desired effect
- **Special Considerations:** Solution is stable for 24 hours at room temperature
  - Discard any solution that is cloudy or discolored or that contains precipitate
- Must be on a cardiac monitor and have continuous BP monitoring for doses above 3 mcg/kg/min

Doxycycline (Vibramycin)

- **Common Adult Dose** >45 kg: 50–200 mg once daily q 12 hours depending on medical disorder
- **Common Child Dose:** ≤45 kg–1.1–4.4 mg/kg once daily q 12 hours depending on medical disorder
- **Reconstitution:** Dilute each 100 mg vial with 10 ml sterile water or 0.9% NaCl
- **Solution Amount:** 100–1000 ml of a compatible solution
- **Compatible Solutions:** D_5W, 0.9% NaCl, D5/LR, Ringer's LR
- **IV Push:** No
- **IVPB:** Yes
- **IV Infusion Time:** Infuse over a minimum of 1–4 hours
- **Special Considerations:** Protect solution from direct sunlight; concentrations <1 mcg/ml or >1 mg/ml not recommended; dilutions with D5/LR or LR must be administered within 6 hours

Droperidol (Inapsine)

- **Common Adult Dose:** 0.5–2.5 mg
- **Common Child Dose:** 0.1 mg/kg
- **Reconstitution:** Administer undiluted
- **Solution Amount:** 250 ml
- **Compatible Solutions:** D₅W, 0.9% NaCl, LR
- **IV Push:** Yes
- **IV Push Rate:** Slowly over 1 minute
- **IVPB:** Yes
- **IV Infusion Time:** Slow IV infusion titrated to patient's response
- **Special Considerations:** High risk for life-threatening cardiac dysrhythmias

Drotrecogin (Xigris)

- **Common Adult Dose:** 24 mcg/kg/hr for 96 hours
- **Common Child Dose:** N/A
- **Reconstitution:** Reconstitute 5 mg vials with 2.5 ml and 20 mg vials with 10 ml sterile water for injection
- **Solution Amount:** Further dilute to a concentration of 100–200 mcg/ml with 0.9% NaCl
- **Compatible Solutions:** 0.9% NaCl, LR, dextrose, and dextrose and saline combinations
- **IV Push:** No
- **IVPB:** Yes
- **IV Infusion Time:** 24 mcg/kg/hr for 96 hours
- **Special Considerations:** Add sterile water to vial slowly; avoid inverting or shaking; gently swirl the vial until powder is dissolved
  - When adding medication to the infusion bag, direct stream to side of the bag to avoid agitating the solution
  - Gently invert bag to mix
  - Solution must be started within 3 hours of mixing and completed within 12 hours
  - Do not administer solution if discolored or if it contains particulate matter

Enalaprilat (Vasotec)

- **Common Adult Dose:** 0.625–1.25 mg every 6 hours
- **Solution Amount:** Dilute in at least 50 ml of fluid
- **Compatible Solutions:** D_5W, 0.9% NaCl, D5/LR
- **IV Push:** Yes
- **IV Push Rate:** May administer undiluted over 5 minutes
- **IVPB:** Yes
- **IV Infusion Time:** Slow infusion
- **Special Considerations:**
  - Diluted solution is stable for 24 hours

Epinephrine (Adrenalin)

- **Common Adult Dose:** 0.1–0.25 mg every 5–15 minutes, followed by an infusion of 1–4 mcg/min as a continuous infusion
- **Common Child Dose:** 0.1 mg; may be followed by a continuous infusion of 0.1–1.5 mcg/kg/min
- **Reconstitution:** Dilute each 1 mg/ml of 1:1000 solution with at least 10 ml of 0.9% NaCl for injection to prepare a 1:10,000 solution
- **Solution Amount:** 250–500 ml
- **Compatible Solutions:** D_5W, 0.9% NaCl
- **IV Push:** Yes
- **IV Push Rate:** Over 1 minute, followed by a 20 ml IV flush
- **IVPB:** Yes
- **IV Infusion Time:** Intermittent infusions can be infused over 5–10 minutes; continuous infusions will be infused at ordered rate
- **Special Considerations:** Must be infused on an infusion pump
- Patient must be on a cardiac monitor and have continuous BP monitoring

Epoetin (Epogen)

- **Common Adult Dose:** 50–150 units/kg 3 times per week
- **Common Child Dose:** 50 units/kg 3 times per week
- **Reconstitution:** Administer undiluted
- **Solution Amount:** N/A
- **Compatible Solutions:** Not specified
- **IV Push:** Yes
- **IVPB:** No
- **IV Push Rate:** Not specified
- **Special Considerations:** Do not shake vial—shaking may inactivate the medication

Eptifibatide (Integrilin)

- **Common Adult Dose:** 135–180 µg/kg as a loading dose; followed by 0.5–2 µg/kg/min
- **Common Child Dose:** N/A
- **Reconstitution:** Administer undiluted
- **Solution Amount:** N/A
- **Compatible Solutions:** N/A—Administer undiluted from the 100 ml vial via an infusion pump
- **IV Push:** Yes
- **IV Push Rate:** Over 1–2 minutes
- **IVPB:** Yes
- **IV Infusion Time:** Based on patient's weight
- **Special Considerations:** Observe patient carefully for indications of bleeding
- Most patients receive heparin and aspirin concurrent with this medication
- Do not administer solution if discolored or if it contains particulate matter

Ergonovine (Ergotrate)

- **Common Adult Dose:** 50–200 mcg every 2–4 hours—maximum of 5 doses
- **Common Child Dose:** N/A
- **Reconstitution:** Dilute with 5 ml of 0.9% NaCl
- **Solution Amount:** N/A
- **Compatible Solutions:** N/A
- **IV Push:** Yes
- **IV Push Rate:** Slowly over 1 minute
- **IVPB:** No
- **Special Considerations:** Giving the medication direct intravenously is reserved for severe uterine bleeding

Ertapenem (Invanz)

- **Common Adult Dose:** 1 g once daily
- **Common Child Dose:** N/A
- **Reconstitution:** Reconstitute with 10 ml of sterile or bacteriostatic water for injection or 0.9% NaCl and shake well
- **Solution Amount:** 50 ml
- **Compatible Solutions:** 0.9% NaCl
- **IV Push:** No
- **IVPB:** Yes
- **IV Infusion Time:** 30 minutes
- **Special Considerations:** Administer within 6 hours after reconstitution
  - Do not administer direct IV
  - Do not infuse with other medications

Erythromycin Gluceptate and Lactobionate (Erythrocin)

- **Common Adult Dose:** 250 mg–1 g every 6 hours
- **Common Child Dose:** 3.75–5 mg/kg every 6 hours

■ **Reconstitution:** Add 10 ml of sterile water for injection without preservatives to 250–500 mg vial; add 20 ml to 1 g vial
■ **Solution Amount:** 100–250 ml
■ **Compatible Solutions:** D$_5$W, 0.9% NaCl
■ **IV Push:** No
■ **IVPB:** Yes
■ **IV Infusion Time:** 20–60 minutes
■ **Special Considerations:** Slow infusion rate if pain occurs along vein during infusion
■ If unable to relieve infusion pain, apply ice and notify physician
■ May infuse as a continuous infusion — 1 g/l of D$_5$W, 0.9% NaCl, or LR over 4 hours

Esmolol (Brevibloc)

■ **Common Adult Dose:** 250–500 mcg loading dose over 1 minute, followed by 50–100 mcg/kg/min infusion; may increase infusion by 50 mcg/kg/min increments until desired effect
■ **Common Child Dose:** 50 mcg/kg/min may be increased every 10 minutes to a maximum of 300 mcg/kg/min
■ **Reconstitution:** 10 mg/ml strength may be administered undiluted
■ **Solution Amount:** Remove 20 ml from a 500 ml bag, and then add 5 g of Esmolol to the bag to make a final concentration of 10 mg/ml
■ **Compatible Solutions:** D$_5$W, D5/0.45% NaCl, D5/0.9% NaCl, 0.9% NaCl, LR, D5/LR
■ **IV Push:** Yes
■ **IV Push Rate:** Loading doses over 1 minute
■ **IVPB:** Yes
■ **IV Infusion Time:** At ordered rate: 50–150 mcg/kg/min
■ **Special Considerations:** Infusions should not be abruptly stopped but tapered off by 25 mcg/kg/min
■ High-alert medication: Have a second practitioner check all doses
■ Must infuse via infusion pump
■ Do not confuse with **Brevital**

Estrogens, Conjugated (Premarin)

- **Common Adult Dose:** 25 mg; may repeat in 6–12 hours if necessary
- **Common Child Dose:** N/A
- **Reconstitution:** Withdraw at least 5 ml of air from the dry container and then slowly introduce the sterile diluent against side of container; gently agitate; do not shake vigorously
- **Solution Amount:** N/A
- **Compatible Solutions:** N/A
- **IV Push:** Yes
- **IV Push Rate:** Slowly over 5 mg/min to prevent flushing
- **IVPB:** No
- **Special Considerations:** Do not use if precipitate is present or if solution is darkened
  - IV is the preferred parenteral route due to the rapid response

Etidronate (Didronel)

- **Common Adult Dose:** 7.5 mg/kg/day for 3 days; may be given as a single dose of 25–30 mg/kg over 24 hours
- **Common Child Dose:** N/A
- **Reconstitution:** N/A
- **Solution Amount:** 250 ml; continuous infusion—1000 ml of 0.9% NaCl
- **Compatible Solutions:** D_5W, 0.9% NaCl
- **IV Push:** No
- **IVPB:** Yes
- **IV Infusion Time:** 2 hours
- **Special Considerations:** May be administered as a continuous infusion over 24 hours

Famotidine (Pepcid)

- **Common Adult Dose:** 20 mg q 12 hours
- **Common Child Dose:** N/A
- **Reconstitution:** N/A
- **Solution Amount:** 100 ml
- **Compatible Solutions:** D_5W, $D_{10}W$, 0.9% NaCl, LR
- **IV Push:** Yes: dilute 2 l of medication in 5–10 ml of 0.9% NaCl
- **IV Push Rate:** Administer over at least 2 minutes
- **IVPB:** Yes
- **IV Infusion Time:** 15–30 minutes
- **Special Considerations:** Do not use solution that is discolored or that contains precipitate

Fenoldopam (Corlopam)

- **Common Adult Dose:** 0.01–1.6 mcg/kg/min
- **Common Child Dose:** N/A
- **Reconstitution:** N/A
- **Solution Amount:** Dilute 40 mg with 1000 ml: 20 mg with 500 ml: 1 mg with 250 ml
- **Compatible Solutions:** D_5W, 0.9% NaCl
- **IV Push:** No—do not use bolus doses
- **IVPB:** Yes
- **IV Infusion Time:** Rate based on body weight
- **Special Considerations:** Must be infused via infusion pump
  - Avoid extravasation
  - Do not admix with other medication
  - Do not administer beta blockers concurrently with this medication

Fentanyl (Sublimaze)

- **Common Adult Dose:** 2–100 mcg/kg
- **Common Child Dose:** 2–3 mcg/kg
- **Reconstitution:** May administer undiluted
- **Solution Amount:** N/A
- **Compatible Solutions:** D_5W, 0.9% NaCl
- **IV Push:** Yes
- **IV Push Rate:** 1–3 minutes
- **IVPB:** Yes
- **IV Infusion Time:** As ordered by physician—may infuse at 25–100 mcg/hr
- **Special Considerations:** Patients receiving this medication must be under care of a practitioner who can manage an airway emergently and who has access to life-support equipment

Filgrastim (Neupogen)

- **Common Adult Dose:** 5 μg/kg/day; may be increased by 5 μg/kg/day with each cycle of chemotherapy
- **Common Child Dose:** N/A
- **Reconstitution:** N/A
- **Solution Amount:** Mix with D_5W to create a final concentration of >15 mcg/ml
- **Compatible Solutions:** D_5W
- **IV Push:** No
- **IVPB:** Yes
- **IV Infusion Time:** 15–30 minutes after chemotherapy; after bone marrow transplant infuse over 4–24 hours
- **Special Considerations:** If infusion concentration is less than 15 mcg/ml, human albumin must be added to the D_5W before the drug is added to the bag
  - Do not freeze the solution
  - May warm to room temperature for up to 6 hours before injection

Fluconazole (Diflucan)

- **Common Adult Dose:** 50–400 mg q day to maximum of 400 mg/day
- **Common Child Dose:** 3–12 mg/kg/day
- **Reconstitution:** Solution comes mixed from manufacturer
- **Compatible Solutions:** D5W, D10W, D5/0.25% NaCl, D5/0.45% NaCl, D5/0.9% NaCl, 0.9% NaCl, LR, D5/LR
- **IV Push:** No
- **IVPB:** Yes
- **IV Infusion Time:** 200 mg/hr
- **Special Considerations:** Do not confuse with **Diprivan**
  - Infusion may have slight opacity, which will diminish gradually
  - Do not administer if solution is cloudy or has precipitate

Flumazenil (Romazicon)

- **Common Adult Dose:** 0.2 mg—may repeat every 1 minute until desired effect
- **Common Child Dose:** 0.01–0.02 mg/kg—may repeat doses of 0.01 mg every 60 seconds times 4 until desired effect achieved
- **Reconstitution:** May be administered undiluted—may be diluted with D5W, or LR if desired
- **Solution Amount:** N/A
- **Compatible Solutions:** N/A
- **IV Push:** Yes
- **IV Push Rate:** 15–30 seconds
- **IVPB:** Yes
- **Special Considerations:** Discard any diluted solution after 24 hours

Folic Acid (Folate)

- **Common Adult and Child Dose:** 0.1–1 mg/day
- **Reconstitution:** May be administered undiluted
- **Solution Amount:** N/A
- **Compatible Solutions:** N/A
- **IV Push:** Yes
- **IV Push Rate:** 5 mg over at least 1 minute
- **IVPB:** Yes: added to hyperalimentation
- **IV Infusion Time:** Added to hyperalimentation

Foscarnet (Foscavir)

- **Common Adult Dose:** 40–90 mg/kg q 8–12 hours, then 90–120 mg/kg/day
- **Common Child Dose:** N/A
- **Reconstitution:** Dilute to 12 mg/ml for a peripheral IV line and 24 mg/ml for a central line
- **Solution Amount:** Dilution as indicated above
- **Compatible Solutions:** D_5W, 0.9% NaCl
- **IV Push:** No
- **IVPB:** Yes
- **IV Infusion Time:** Administer at a rate of 1 mg/kg/min; maintenance dose can be infused over 2 hours
- **Special Considerations:** Infuse on an infusion pump

Fosphenytoin (Cerebyx)

- **Common Adult Dose:** 5–20 mg PE/kg (loading); 4–6 mg PE/kg/day (maintenance)
- **Common Child Dose:** 5–20 mg PE/kg (loading); 4–6 mg PE/kg/day (maintenance)
- **Reconstitution:** N/A
- **Solution Amount:** Dilute to a concentration of 1.5–25 mg PE/ml
- **Compatible Solutions:** D_5W, 0.9% NaCl
- **IV Push:** Yes

- **IV Push Rate:** <150 mg PE/min to reduce risk of hypotension
- **IVPB:** No
- **Special Considerations:** May be refrigerated for up to 48 hours

Furosemide (Lasix)

- **Common Adult Dose:** 20–100 mg
- **Common Child Dose:** 1 mg/kg; may increase by 1 mg/kg every 2 hours until desired effect
- **Reconstitution:** Can administer undiluted; may dilute large doses
- **Solution Amount:** Not specified
- **Compatible Solutions:** D₅W, D₁₀W, D₂₀W, D5/0.9% NaCl, 0.9% NaCl, LR, D5/LR, 3% NaCl, 1/6 M sodium lactate
- **IV Push:** Yes
- **IV Push Rate:** 10–20 mg/min
- **IVPB:** Yes
- **IV Infusion Time:** Do not exceed 4 mg/min
- **Special Considerations:** Use an infusion pump for intermittent infusions

Ganciclovir (Cytovene)

- **Common Adult Dose:** 5–6 mg/kg every 12–24 hours
- **Common Child Dose:** N/A
- **Reconstitution:** Reconstitute 500 mg with 10 ml of sterile water (do not use bacteriostatic agents)
- **Solution Amount:** 100 ml
- **Compatible Solutions:** D₅W, 0.9% NaCl, LR, Ringer's solution
- **IV Push:** No
- **IVPB:** Yes
- **IV Infusion Time:** Slowly over 1 hour, using an infusion pump
- **Special Considerations:** Wear gowns, gloves, and mask while handling medication
  - ■ Discard IV equipment in specially designed containers
  - ■ Discard medication if discoloration or particulate matter is evident

Gatifloxacin (Tequin)

- **Common Adult Dose**: 400 mg every 24 hours
- **Common Child Dose**: N/A
- **Reconstitution**: Dilute to a concentration of 2 mg/ml
- **Solution Amount**: Dilute to a concentration of 2 mg/2 ml
- **Compatible Solutions**: D5W, D5/0.9% NaCl, 0.9% NaCl, D5/LR
- **IV Push**: No
- **IVPB**: Yes
- **IV Infusion Time**: 60 minutes
- **Special Considerations**: Avoid rapid infusion

Gentamicin (Garamycin)

- **Common Adult Dose**: Maximum of 5 mg/kg/day in 3–4 divided doses
- **Common Child Dose**: 2–2.5 mg/kg every 8 hours
- **Reconstitution**: N/A
- **Solution Amount**: 50–200 ml (do not exceed concentration of 1 mg/ml)
- **Compatible Solutions**: D5W, 0.9% NaCl, LR
- **IV Push**: No
- **IVPB**: Yes
- **Infusion Time**: 30 minutes to 2 hours
- **Special Considerations**: Do not infuse solutions that are discolored or that contain precipitate

Glucagon (GlucaGen)

- **Common Adult Dose**: 1 mg; may repeat in 15 minutes if needed
- **Common Child Dose**: 20–30 mcg; may be repeated in 15 minutes if needed
- **Reconstitution**: Use diluent supplied with medication unless giving a dose >2 mg, then use sterile water to decrease the risk of thrombophlebitis (final concentration should not exceed 1 mg/ml)
- **Solution Amount**: N/A
- **Compatible Solutions**: N/A

- **IV Push:** Yes
- **IV Push Rate:** 1 mg/min
- **IVPB:** No
- **Special Considerations:** Stable for 48 hours if refrigerated

Glycopyrrolate (Robinul)

- **Common Adult Dose:** 100–200 µg; may repeat every 2–3 minutes
- **Common Child Dose:** 4.4 µg/kg up to 100 mcg; may be repeated every 2–3 minutes
- **Reconstitution:** Give undiluted
- **Compatible Solutions:** D$_5$W, D5/0.45 NaCl, 0.9% NaCl, Ringer's
- **IV Push:** Yes
- **IV Push Rate:** 0.2 mg over 1–2 minutes
- **IVPB:** No

Granisetron (Kytril)

- **Common Adult and Child Dose:** 10 mcg/kg
- **Reconstitution:** May be administered
- **Solution Amount:** May dilute in 20–50 ml
- **Compatible Solutions:** D$_5$W, 0.9% NaCl
- **IV Push:** Yes
- **IV Push Rate:** Undiluted over 30 seconds; diluted over 5 minutes
- **IVPB:** No

Haloperidol (Haldol)

- **Common Adult Dose:** 0.5–5 mg; may repeat every 30 minutes
- **Common Child Dose:** N/A
- **Reconstitution:** May be administered undiluted
- **Solution Amount:** 30–50 ml
- **Compatible Solutions:** D$_5$W
- **IV Push:** Yes
- **IV Push Rate:** 5 mg/min
- **IVPB:** Yes
- **IV Infusion Time:** 30 minutes

Heparin (Heparin)

- **Common Adult Dose:** 10,000 U bolus followed by 5000–10,000 q 4–6 hours; continuous infusion of 20,000–40,000 units infused over 24 hours
- **Common Child Dose:** 50 U/kg bolus followed by 50–100 U/kg q 4 hours
- **Reconstitution:** May be administered undiluted
- **Solution Amount:** Prescribed amount—typically 500 ml
- **Compatible Solutions:** D_5W, 0.9% NaCl, Ringer's
- **IV Push:** Yes
- **IV Push Rate:** Over at least 1 minute
- **IVPB:** Yes: continuous infusion
- **IV Infusion Time:** Prescribed rate—usually over 4–24 hours
- **Special Considerations:** Continuous infusions must be placed on an infusion pump

Hydralazine (Apresoline)

- **Common Adult Dose:** 5–40 mg repeated as needed
- **Common Child Dose:** 1.7–3.5 mg/kg/day in 4–6 divided doses
- **Reconstitution:** N/A
- **Compatible Solutions:** D_5W, $D_{10}W$, D5/0.25% NaCl, D5/0.45% NaCl, D5/0.9% NaCl, 0.9% NaCl, LR, D5/LR
- **IV Push:** Yes; administer undiluted
- **IV Push Rate:** Administer at a rate of 10 mg over at least 1 minute
- **IVPB:** N/A
- **IV Infusion Time:** N/A
- **Special Considerations:** Administer as quickly as possible after drawing through a filter needle into a syringe; hydralazine changes color after contact with a metal filter

Hydrocortisone Sodium Phosphate
(Solu-Cortef & Cortef)

- **Common Adult Dose:** 100–500 mg every 2–6 hours
- **Common Child Dose:** 0.186–0.28 mg/kg/day in 3 divided doses
- **Reconstitution:** Reconstitute with provided solution or with 2 ml of bacteriostatic water or saline for injection
- **Solution Amount:** 50–1000 ml
- **Compatible Solutions:** D$_5$W, D5/0.9% NaCl, 0.9% NaCl
- **IV Push:** Yes
- **IV Push Rate:** Administer each 100 mg over at least 30 seconds; doses of 500 mg or greater should be infused over at least 10 minutes
- **IVPB:** Yes
- **IV Infusion Time:** Not specified
- **Special Considerations:** Diluted solutions should be infused within 24 hours

Hydrocortisone Sodium Succinate
(Solu-Cortef & Cortef)

- **Common Adult Dose:** 100–500 mg every 2–6 hours
- **Common Child Dose:** 0.186–0.28 mg/kg/day in 3 divided doses
- **Reconstitution:** Reconstitute with provided solution or with 2 ml of bacteriostatic water or saline for injection
- **Solution Amount:** 50–1000 ml
- **Compatible Solutions:** D$_5$W, D5/0.9% NaCl, 0.9% NaCl
- **IV Push:** Yes
- **IV Push Rate:** Administer each 100 mg over at least 30 seconds; doses of 500 mg or greater should be infused over at least 10 minutes
- **IVPB:** Yes
- **IV Infusion Time:** Not specified
- **Special Considerations:** Diluted solutions should be infused within 24 hours

Hydromorphone (Dilaudid)

- **Common Adult Dose:** 1.5 mg q 3–4 hours as needed; continuous infusion: 0.2–30 mg/hr
- **Common Child Dose:** 0.015 mg/kg every 3–4 hours as needed
- **Reconstitution:** N/A
- **Solution Amount:** N/A
- **Compatible Solutions:** D_5W, D5/0.45% NaCl, D5/0.9% NaCl, 0.45% NaCl, 0.9% NaCl, LR, D5/LR, Ringer's
- **IV Push:** Yes; dilute with at least 5 ml of sterile water or 0.9% NaCl for injection
- **IV Push Rate:** At a rate not to exceed 2 mg over 3–5 minutes
- **IVPB:** No
- **IV Infusion Time:** N/A
- **Special Considerations:** Slight yellow coloration does not alter potency; inspect for particulate matter

HOT TIP: Hydroxyzine (Vistaril) cannot be given intravenously!

Hyoscyamine (Levsin)

- **Common Adult Dose:** 0.125–0.5 mg 3–4 times daily
- **Common Child Dose:** 0.0005 mg/kg preoperatively
- **IV Push:** Yes; give undiluted or diluted in 10 ml of sterile water
- **IV Push Rate:** Not specified
- **IVPB:** No

Ibutilide (Corvert)

- **Common Adult Dose:** 0.005 mg/kg infusion; may be repeated once (smaller dose given following cardiac surgery)
- **Common Child Dose:** N/A
- **Reconstitution:** N/A
- **Solution Amount:** 50 ml
- **Compatible Solutions:** D_5W, 0.9% NaCl
- **IV Push:** No

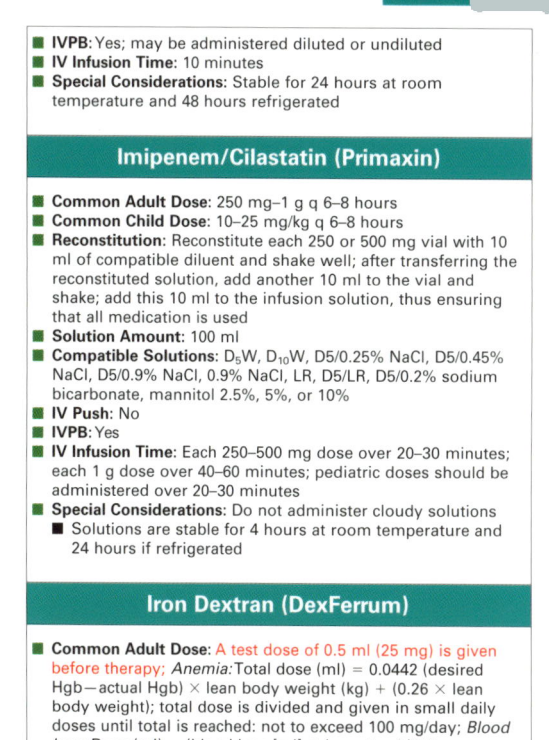

- **IVPB:** Yes; may be administered diluted or undiluted
- **IV Infusion Time:** 10 minutes
- **Special Considerations:** Stable for 24 hours at room temperature and 48 hours refrigerated

Imipenem/Cilastatin (Primaxin)

- **Common Adult Dose:** 250 mg–1 g q 6–8 hours
- **Common Child Dose:** 10–25 mg/kg q 6–8 hours
- **Reconstitution:** Reconstitute each 250 or 500 mg vial with 10 ml of compatible diluent and shake well; after transferring the reconstituted solution, add another 10 ml to the vial and shake; add this 10 ml to the infusion solution, thus ensuring that all medication is used
- **Solution Amount:** 100 ml
- **Compatible Solutions:** D_5W, $D_{10}W$, D5/0.25% NaCl, D5/0.45% NaCl, D5/0.9% NaCl, 0.9% NaCl, LR, D5/LR, D5/0.2% sodium bicarbonate, mannitol 2.5%, 5%, or 10%
- **IV Push:** No
- **IVPB:** Yes
- **IV Infusion Time:** Each 250–500 mg dose over 20–30 minutes; each 1 g dose over 40–60 minutes; pediatric doses should be administered over 20–30 minutes
- **Special Considerations:** Do not administer cloudy solutions
  - Solutions are stable for 4 hours at room temperature and 24 hours if refrigerated

Iron Dextran (DexFerrum)

- **Common Adult Dose:** A test dose of 0.5 ml (25 mg) is given before therapy; *Anemia:* Total dose (ml) = 0.0442 (desired Hgb—actual Hgb) × lean body weight (kg) + (0.26 × lean body weight); total dose is divided and given in small daily doses until total is reached: not to exceed 100 mg/day; *Blood loss:* Dose (ml) = (blood loss [ml] × hematocrit)/50
- **Common Child Dose:** A test dose of 0.5 ml (25 mg) is given before therapy; *Anemia:* Total dose (ml) = 0.0442 (desired

Hgb—actual Hgb) × lean body weight (kg) + (0.26 × lean body weight); total dose is divided and given in small daily doses until total is reached: not to exceed 25 mg/day in children <5 kg and not to exceed 50 mg/day in children <10 kg

- **Reconstitution:** May be administered undiluted
- **Solution Amount:** 200–1000 ml if prepared as an infusion
- **Compatible Solutions:** 0.9% NaCl (preferred), D₅W (related to increased incidences of pain and phlebitis)
- **IV Push:** Yes; may be administered undiluted
- **IV Push Rate:** 50 mg/min
- **IVPB:** Yes
- **IV Infusion Time:** 1–8 hours followed by a test infusion at 10 gtt/min for 10 minutes
- **Special Considerations:** Flush IV line with 10 ml of 0.9% NaCl at the completion of the infusion
  - Can be added to total parenteral nutrition

Iron Sucrose (Venofer)

- **Common Adult Dose:** 100 mg (5 ml) during each dialysis session up to 3 times per week for a total of 10 doses; additional smaller doses may be necessary
- **Common Child Dose:** N/A
- **Reconstitution:** N/A
- **Solution Amount:** 100 ml mixed immediately before administration
- **Compatible Solutions:** 0.9% NaCl
- **IV Push:** Yes; undiluted, directly into dialysis line
- **IV Push Rate:** 1 ml undiluted per minute, not to exceed 1 vial per injection
- **IVPB:** Yes: directly into dialysis line (may reduce risk of hypotension)
- **IV Infusion Time:** At least 15 minutes
- **Special Considerations:** Do not administer iron sucrose concurrently with oral iron as the absorption of oral iron is reduced
  - Do not add to parenteral nutrition solutions

Itraconazole (Sporanox)

- **Common Adult Dose:** 200 mg twice a day for 4 doses, then 200 mg once a day
- **Common Child Dose:** N/A
- **Reconstitution:** N/A
- **Solution Amount:** 50 ml
- **Compatible Solutions:** 0.9% NaCl
- **IV Push:** No
- **IVPB:** Yes
- **IV Infusion Time:** Use an infusion control device and infuse over 60 minutes
- **Special Considerations:** Flush line with 15–20 ml of 0.9% NaCl over 30 seconds to 15 minutes

Kanamycin (Kantrex)

- **Common Adult and Child Dose:** 5–7.5 mg/kg q 8 or q 12 hours
- **Reconstitution:** N/A
- **Solution Amount:** 500 mg: in 100–200 ml; each gram in 200–400 ml (dilute in smaller proportionate volume for children)
- **Compatible Solutions:** D_5W, $D_{10}W$, 0.9% NS, D5/0.9%NaCL, LR
- **IV Push:** No
- **IVPB:** Yes
- **IV Infusion Time:** 30–60 minutes
- **Special Considerations:** Darkening of solution does not alter potency

Ketorolac (Toradol)

- **Common Adult Dose:** 15–30 mg q 6 hours (lower dose is used for adults >65 years old or with renal impairment)
- **Common Child Dose:** N/A
- **Reconstitution:** N/A

- **Compatible Solutions:** D$_5$W, D5/0.9% NaCl, 0.9% NaCl, LR, Ringer's injection
- **IV Push:** Yes
- **IV Push Rate:** Undiluted over at least 15 seconds
- **IVPB:** No
- **IV Push Rate:** Undiluted, over at least 15 seconds
- **Special Considerations:** Should be discontinued after 5 days of administration by all routes

Labetalol (Normodyne)

- **Common Adult Dose:** 20 mg initially followed by additional doses of 40–80 mg as needed every 10 minutes, not to exceed 300 mg total dose; may be administered as an infusion of 2 mg/min with a range of 50–300 mg total dose
- **Common Child Dose:** N/A
- **Reconstitution:** N/A
- **Solution Amount:** Add 200 mg to 160 ml of solution for a final concentration of 1 mg/ml or 200 mg to 250 ml of solution for a final concentration of 2 mg/3 ml
- **Compatible Solutions:** D$_5$W, D5/0.25% NaCl, D5/0.9% NaCl, 0.9% NaCl, LR, D5/LR
- **IV Push:** Yes, undiluted
- **IV Push Rate:** slowly over 2 minutes
- **IVPB:** Yes
- **IV Infusion Time:** Infuse via an infusion pump starting at 2 mg/min and titrating up to desired effect
- **Special Considerations:** Do not confuse with **Lamictal**
- Continuous BP monitoring is required

Lepirudin (Refludan)

- **Common Adult Dose:** 0.4 mg/kg (not to exceed 44 mg) as a bolus, followed by 0.15 mg/kg/hr (not to exceed 16.5 mg/hr) initially; subsequent adjustments made on the basis of aPTT but should not exceed infusion rate of 0.21 mg/kg/hr without checking for coagulation abnormalities

- **Common Child Dose:** N/A
- **Reconstitution:** 1 ml of sterile water for injection or 0.9% NaCl; shake gently; clear, colorless solution should be obtained within a few seconds to 3 minutes; for infusion reconstitute 2 vials with 1 ml each of sterile water for injection or 0.9% NaCl
- **Solution Amount:** Add reconstituted solution to a 10 ml syringe and dilute to a total of 10 ml; 250–500 ml of D_5W or 0.9% NaCl
- **Compatible Solutions:** D_5W, 0.9% NaCl, sterile water for injection (for reconstitution)
- **IV Push:** Yes
- **IV Push Rate:** Slowly over 15–20 minutes
- **IVPB:** Yes
- **IV Infusion Time:** Infuse at 0.15 mg/kg/hr using an infusion pump
- **Special Considerations:** Warm to room temperature before administering
  - Do not admix with other drugs

Levofloxacin (Levaquin)

- **Common Adult Dose:** 250–750 mg q 24 hours
- **Common Child Dose:** N/A
- **Reconstitution:** Dilute to a concentration of 5 mg/ml
- **Solution Amount:** Dilute to a concentration of 5 mg/ml
- **Compatible Solutions:** D_5W, $D_{10}10$, D5, D5/0.45% NaCl, D5/0.9% NaCl, 0.9% NaCl, D5/LR, 5% sodium bicarbonate, D5, Plasmalyte 56, sodium lactate
- **IV Push:** No
- **IVPB:** Yes
- **IV Infusion Time:** 60 minutes
- **Special Considerations:** Avoid rapid infusion

Lidocaine (Parenteral)

- **Common Adult Dose:** 50–100 mg (1 mg/kg) bolus (may be repeated in 5 minutes), then 1–4 mg/min (20–50 μg/kg/min) infusion (up to 4.5 mg/kg or 300 mg in 1 hour)
- **Common Child Dose:** 1 mg/kg bolus; may be repeated after 5 minutes (not to exceed 3 mg/kg), followed by 30 mcg/kg/min infusion (range 20–50 mcg/kg/min)
- **Reconstitution:** Not specified
- **Solution Amount:** Only 1% and 2% solutions are used for direct IV injection
- **Compatible Solutions:** D₅W, D5/LR, 0.45% NaCl, D5/0.9% NaCl, D5/0.45% NaCl, 0.9% NaCl, LR
- **IV Push:** Yes: administer undiluted IV loading dose of 1 mg/kg
- **IV Push Rate:** 25–50 mg over 1 minute; may repeat dose after 5 minutes, followed by IV infusion
- **IVPB:** Yes: to prepare add 1 g lidocaine to 250, 500, or 1000 ml of a compatible solution; solution is stable for 24 hours
- **IVPB Infusion:** Administer via infusion pump for accurate dose at a rate of 1–4 mg/min
- **Special Considerations:** Do not use lidocaine with preservatives or other medications, such as epinephrine, for IV infusion
- Requires cardiac monitoring

Linezolid (Zyvox)

- **Common Adult Dose:** 400–600 mg every 12 hours for 10–28 days
- **Common Child Dose:** 10 mg/kg every 8–12 hours for 10–14 days
- **Reconstitution:** Injection is administered in single and ready-to-use infusion bags; do not administer infusion containing particulate matter
- **Compatible Solutions:** D5/0.45% NaCl, D5/09% NaCl, D₅W, 0.9% NaCl LR
- **IV Push:** No
- **IVPB Infusion:** Administer over 30–120 minutes; flush line before and after use
- **Special Considerations:** Do not use bag in series connections

Liothyronine (Cytomel, T3)

- **Common Adult Dose:** 25-50 mcg initially (see special considerations); may give additional doses not to exceed 100 µg/day; doses should be at least 4 hours apart and not more than 12 hours apart
- **Solution Amount:** Give undiluted
- **Compatible Solutions:** Unavailable
- **IV Push:** Yes; undiluted
- **IV Push Rate:** Bolus—1 minute
- **Special Considerations:** For IV only—not for intramuscular or subcutaneous injection; in case of cardiovascular disease, initial dose should be 10-20 mcg

Lorazepam (Ativan)

- **Common Adult Dose:** *Preoperative sedation* (not to exceed 2 mg) 15-20 minutes before surgery. *Antiemetic* (2 mg) 30 minutes before chemotherapy; may be repeated q 4 hours, as needed). *Anticonvulsant:* 50 mcg/kg, up to 4 mg; may be repeated after 10-15 minutes (not to exceed 8 mg/12 hr [unlabeled])
- **Reconstitution:** Dilute immediately before use with an equal amount of sterile water, D₅W, or 0.9% NaCl for injection; do not use if solution is colored or contains a precipitate
- **Solution Amount:** 1-2 mg/ml
- **Compatible Solutions:** 0.9% NaCl, D₅W
- **IV Push:** Yes; administer direct IV through Y-site
- **IV Push Rate:** 2 mg over 1 minute
- **IVPB Infusion:** No
- **Special Considerations:** Rapid IV administration may result in apnea, hypotension, bradycardia, or cardiac arrest

Magnesium Sulfate (9/9% mg; 8.1 mEq mg/g)

- **Common Adult Dose:** *Severe deficiency* (5 g), *Eclampsia/pre-eclampsia* (4–5 g by IV infusion, concurrently with up to 5 g IM in each buttock; then 4–5 g IM q 4 hours *or* 4 g by IV infusion followed by 1–2 g/hr continuous infusion; not to exceed 40 g/day or 20 g/48 hr in the presence of severe renal insufficiency); *Part of Parenteral Nutrition* 4–24 mEq day
- **Common Child Dose:** *Part of Parenteral Nutrition* 0.25–0.5 mEq/day
- **Reconstitution:** (see IV push and IVPB)
- **Compatible Solutions:** (see IV push and IVPB)
- **IV Push:** Yes: administer 10% solution undiluted
- **IV Push Rate:** 1.5 ml (or its equivalent) over 1 minute
- **IVPB:** Yes: *anticonvulsant* (dilute 4 g in 250 ml of D_5W or 0.9% NaCl and administer at a rate not to exceed 3 ml/min); *Hypomagnesemia* (dilute 5 g in 1000 ml of D_5W, 0.9% NaCl, or Ringer's or LR and administer slowly over 3 hours)
- **Special Considerations:** For IVPB, use infusion pump to regulate rate accurately. Accidental overdosage of IV magnesium has resulted in serious patient harm as well as death. Have a second practitioner independently double-check original order, dosage calculation, and infusion pump settings

Mannitol (Osmitrol)

- **Common Adult Dose:** *Edema, oliguric renal failure:* 50–100 g as a 5%–25% solution; may precede with a test dose of 0.2 g/kg over 3–5 minutes; *Reduction of intracranial/intraocular pressure:* 0.25–2g/kg as 15%–25% solutions over 30–60 minutes; *Diuresis in drug intoxications:* 50–200 g as a 5%–25% solution titrated to maintain urine flow of 100–500 ml/hr
- **Common Child Dose:** *Edema, oliguric renal failure:* 0.25–2g/kg (60 g/m^2) as a 15%–20% solution over 2–6 hours; may precede with a test dose of 0.2 g/kg over 3–5 minutes; *Reduction of intracranial/intraocular pressure:* 1–2 g/kg (30–60 g/m^2) as a 15%–20% solution over 30–60 minutes; *Diuresis in drug intoxications:* up to 2 g/kg (60 g/m^2) as a 5%–10% solution

Reconstitution: Administer by IV infusion undiluted

■ **IV Push:** Yes
■ **IV Push Rate:** Test Dose—administer over 3-5 minutes for urine output of 30-50 ml/hr; if urine output does not increase, administer a second test dose; if urine output is not at least 30-50 ml/hr for 2-3 hours after second test dose, patient should be reevaluated
■ **IV Push Rate:** Slowly, over 15-20 minutes
  ■ If oliguria, rate should be titrated to produce a urine output of 30-50 ml/hr; child's dose over 2-6 hours
  ■ If intracranial pressure, infuse dose over 30-60 minutes in adults and children
  ■ If intraocular pressure, administer dose over 30 minutes
  ■ If preoperative, administer 60-90 minutes
  ■ If for irrigation, add contents of two 50 ml vials of 25% mannitol to 900 ml of sterile water for injection of a 2.5% solution
■ **IVPB:** No
■ **Special Considerations:** If solution contains crystals, warm bottle in hot water and shake vigorously; do not administer if all crystals are not dissolved; cool to body temperature; use an in-line filter for 15%, 20%, and 25% solutions

Melphalan (Alkeran)

■ **Common Adult Dose:** 16 mg/m² q 2 weeks for 4 doses, then q 4 weeks
■ **Reconstitution:** Reconstitute with 10 ml of supplied diluent—concentration of 5 mg/ml and shake vigorously until clear; dilute immediately with 0.9% NaCl for a concentration of ≤0.45 mg/ml; must administer within 60 minutes of reconstitution
■ **Compatible Solutions:** Supplied diluent
■ **IV Push:** No
■ **IVPB:** Yes: see above
■ **Infusion Time:** Over at least 15 minutes; IVPB
■ **Special Considerations:** Monitor complete blood count, liver function tests, uric acid during therapy

Meperidine (Demerol)

- **Common Adult Dose**: 15–35 mg/hr continuous infusion. *PCA:* 10 mg at first, with a range of 1–5 mg increments; lockout interval recommended is 6–10 minutes with a minimum of 5 minutes
- **Common Child Dose**: N/A
- **Compatible Solutions**: For IVPB: D_5W, $D_{10}W$, dextrose/saline combinations, dextrose/Ringer's or lactated Ringer's injection combinations, 0.45% NaCl, 0.9% NaCl, or Ringer's or LR
- **IV Push**: Yes: dilute to a concentration of 10 mg/ml
- **IV Push Rate**: IV push slowly. Rapid administration can lead to hypotension, respiratory depression, and circulatory collapse
- **IVPB**: Yes: dilute to a concentration of 1 mg/ml
- **Special Considerations**: Infusion must be by IV pump

Methocarbamol (Robaxin)

- **Common Adult Dose**: 1–3 g/day for not more than 3 days; course may be repeated after a 48-hour rest
- **Compatible Solutions**: 0.9% NaCl, D_5W
- **IV Push**: Yes: administer undiluted at a rate of 3 ml (300 mg)
- **IV Push Rate**: Over 1 minute
- **IVPB**: Yes: dilute each dose in no more than 250 ml of a compatible solution
- **Infusion Time**: Not specified
- **Special Considerations**: Patient should remain recumbent during and at least 10–15 minutes after infusion to avoid orthostatic hypotension

Methotrexate (Amethopterin, Folex)

- **Common Adult Dose**: Range of 5 mg to 12 g for a variety of disorders; see literature for specific dose for each disorder
- **Reconstitution**: For IV Push—reconstitute each vial with 25 ml of 0.9% NaCl—concentration no greater than 25 mg/ml

- **Compatible Solutions:** 0.9% NaCl
- **IV Push:** Yes
- **IV Push Rate:** 10 mg/min
- **IVPB:** Yes
- **IVPB Infusion Time:** 4–20 mg/hr as continuous or intermittent infusion
- **Compatible Solutions:** D₅W, D5/0.9% NaCl, or 0.9% NaCl
- **Special Considerations:** Use sterile preservative-free diluents for high-dose regimens; reconstitute immediately before use—discard unused portion

Methyldopa (Aldomet)

- **Common Adult Dose:** 250–500 mg q 6 hours up to 1 g q 6 hours
- **Common Child Dose:** 5–10 mg/kg q 6 h given up to 65 mg/kg/day in divided doses (do not exceed 3 g daily)
- **Solution Amount:** 100 ml
- **Compatible Solutions:** 0.9% NaCl, D₅W, D5/0.9% NaCl, 5% sodium bicarbonate, or Ringer's solution
- **IV Push:** No
- **IVPB:** Yes
- **Infusion Time:** Infuse slowly over 30–60 minutes
- **Special Considerations:** Monitor BP and pulse frequently

Methylergonovine (Methergine)

- **Common Adult Dose:** 200 µg (0.2 mg) q 2–4 hours for up to 5 doses
- **Common Child Dose:** N/A
- **Compatible Solutions:** 0.9% NaCl
- **IV Push:** Yes; can be given undiluted or diluted in 5 ml of 0.9% NaCl
- **IV Push Rate:** 0.2 mg over at least 1 minute
- **IVPB:** No
- **Special Considerations:** IV administration is used for emergencies only; do not add to IV solutions or mix in a syringe with any other drug

Methylprednisolone (Solu-Medrol)

- **Common Adult Dose:** 10–40 mg repeated as needed
- **Common Child Dose:** 117 mcg/kg in 3 divided doses; 139–835 mcg/kg every 12–24 hours
- **Reconstitution:** Reconstitute with provided diluent or 2 ml of bacteriostatic water for injection
- **Solution Amount:** Not specified
- **Compatible Solutions:** D_5W, D5/0.9% NaCl, 0.9% NaCl
- **IV Push:** Yes
- **IV Push Rate:** Over 1 to several minutes
- **IVPB:** Yes
- **IV Infusion Time:** May be infused at ordered rate or as a continuous infusion at ordered rate
- **Special Considerations:** Solution may form a haze upon dilution

Metoclopramide (Reglan)

- **Common Adult Dose:** *Prevention of chemo-induced N/V:* 1/2 mg/kg every 30 minutes before chemo administration; additional doses may be given—see the literature
- **Common Child Dose:** 2.5–5 mg; <6 years: 0.1 mg/kg
- **Compatible Solutions:** D_5W, 0.9% NaCl, D5/0.45% NaCl, Ringer's solution, or LR
- **IV Push:** Yes
- **IV Push Rate:** 1–2 minutes, 30 minutes before chemotherapy
- **IVPB:** May be diluted with 50 ml of a compatible solution
- **IVPB Infusion Time:** Infuse slowly over at least 15 minutes
- **Special Considerations:** Too rapid administration causes transient, but intense, feeling of anxiety and restlessness, followed by drowsiness

Metoprolol (Lopressor)

- **Common Adult Dose:** 5 mg q 2 minutes for 3 doses, followed by oral dosing
- **Common Child Dose:** N/A
- **Compatible Solutions:** Not specified
- **IV Push:** Yes
- **IV Push Rate:** Rapidly at 2-minute intervals
- **IVPB:** Yes

Metronidazole (Flagyl)

- **Common Adult Dose:** 500 mg–750 mg q 6–8 hours
- **Common Child Dose:** N/A
- **Reconstitution:** Add 4.4 ml of sterile water, sterile bacteriostatic water, 0.9% NaCl for injection
- **Compatible Solutions:** 0.9% NaCl, D5W, LR
- **Solution Amount:** 100 mg/ml
- **IV Push:** No
- **IVPB:** Yes; dilute to at least 8 mg/ml with a compatible solution; neutralize solution with 5 mEq sodium bicarbonate for each 500 mg
- **Infusion Time:** Infuse each dose slowly over 1 hour
- **Special Considerations:** Do not use aluminum needles or hubs—color will turn orange/rust

Midazolam (Versed)

- **Common Adult Dose:** 1–1.5 mg initially, dose increased as needed; total dose >5 mg rarely needed; as an infusion: 20–100 mcg/kg/hr
- **Common Child Dose:** 25–100 mcg/kg, not to exceed 10 mg total; as an infusion: 30–120 mcg/kg/min
- **Reconstitution:** N/A
- **Solution Amount:** Dilute 5 mg/min to a concentration of 0.5 mg/ml with D5W or 0.9% NaCl
- **Compatible Solutions:** D5W, 0.9% NaCl, LR

- **IV Push:** Yes, diluted or undiluted
- **IV Push Rate:** Slowly over 2 minutes
- **IVPB:** Yes, as an infusion
- **IV Infusion Time:** Titrate to desired level of sedation: 1–7 mg/hr for adults and 0.5–2 mcg/kg/min for children
- **Special Considerations:** Do not confuse with **VePesid**
- Patient must be on a cardiac monitor and pulse oximeter; conscious sedation principles apply

Milrinone (Primacor) High Alert

- **Common Adult Dose:** *Loading dose:* 50 mcg/kg followed by *infusion* at 0.05 mcg/kg/min
- **Common Child Dose:** N/A
- **Reconstitution:** Dilute a 20 mg vial with 180 ml of a compatible solution for a concentration of 100 mcg/ml; 113 ml of a compatible solution for a concentration of 150 mcg/ml; 80 ml of a compatible solution for a concentration of 200 mcg/ml
- **Compatible Solutions:** 0.9% NaCl, 0.45% NaCl, D₅W
- **IV Push:** Yes: loading dose may be given undiluted
- **IV Push Rate:** Over 10 minutes
- **IVPB:** Yes
- **Infusion Time:** Infusion rate is titrated according to hemodynamic and clinical response—see reconstitution
- **Special Considerations:** Accidental overdose can cause patient harm or death; have another practitioner check order, calculation of dose, and infusion settings

Minocycline (Minocin, Vectrin)

- **Common Adult Dose:** Initially 200 mg, then 100 mg q 12 hours up to 400 mg/day
- **Common Child Dose:** ≥8 years—initially 4 mg/kg, then 2 mg/kg q 12 hours
- **Reconstitution:** Dilute a 100 mg vial with 5–10 ml sterile water
- **Solution Amount:** 500–1000 ml of a compatible solution
- **Compatible Solutions:** D₅W, D5/0.9% NaCl, Ringer's solution, LR
- **IV Push:** No

- **IVPB:** Yes
- **IV Infusion Time:** Infuse immediately following dilution over 6 hours
- **Special Considerations:** If given rapidly, may cause thrombophlebitis; observe for signs of extravasation throughout infusion

Morphine

- **Common Adult Dose:** (≥50 kg) pain; 4–10 mg q 3–4 hours; MI/8–15 mg; (≤50 kg) pain: 0.1 mg/kg q 3–4 hours. Continuous infusion: 0.8–10 mg/hr
- **Common Child Dose:** (≤50 kg) pain; 0.1 mg/kg q 3–4 hours
- **Compatible Solutions:** D_5W, $D_{10}W$, 0.9% NaCl, 0.45% NaCl, Ringer's, LR
- **IV Push:** Yes: dilute with at least 5 ml of sterile water or 0.9% NaCl
- **IV Push Rate:** 2.5–15 mg over 4–5 minutes
- **IV Continuous Infusion:** Yes: add to a compatible solution at a concentration of 0.1–1 mg/ml or greater
- **Infusion Time:** Administer via an infusion or PCA pump; titrate dose to ensure adequate pain relief without excessive sedation, respiratory depression, and hypotension
- **Special Considerations:** Rapid administration may lead to increased respiratory depression, hypotension, and circulatory collapse

Moxifloxacin (Avelox)

- **Common Adult Dose:** 400 mg/day
- **Common Child Dose:** N/A
- **Reconstitution:** Premixed bags should not be further diluted
- **Solution Amount:** N/A
- **Compatible Solutions:** D_5W, $D_{10}W$, 0.9% NaCl, LR
- **IV Push:** No
- **IVPB:** Yes
- **IV Infusion Time:** 60 minutes
- **Special Considerations:** Avoid rapid or bolus infusion

Muromonab-CD3 (Orthoclone OKT3)

- **Common Adult Dose:** 5 mg/day for 10–14 days
- **Common Child Dose:** (100 mcg) 0.1 mg/kg/day for 10–14 days
- **Compatible Solutions:** 0.9% NaCl—Do not admix or administer in line with other medications
- **IV Push:** Yes
- **IV Push Rate:** Administer <1 minute; use a 0.2 or 0.22 micrometer filter to draw up solution into syringe; remove filter needle, and attach a 20 g needle for IV administration
- **IVPB:** No
- **Special Considerations:** Do not administer as an infusion

Mycophenolate (CellCept)

- **Common Adult Dose:** 1 g–1.5 g twice daily, depending on transplantation type
- **Reconstitution:** Reconstitute each vial with 14 ml D_5W; shake gently to dissolve—solution will be slightly yellow
- **Compatible Solutions:** D_5W—do not admix or administer in same tubing as other medications
- **IV Push:** No
- **IVPB:** Yes: dilute contents of 2 vials (1 g dose) with 140 ml of D_5W; 3 vials (1.5 g dose) with 210 ml of D_5W—concentration 6 mg/ml
- **Infusion Time:** Administer slowly over 2 hours
- **Special Considerations:** IV route should be used only for patients unable to take oral medications

Nalbuphine (Nubain)

- **Common Adult Dose:** 10 mg q 3–6 hours (do not exceed 20 mg single dose or daily dose of 160 mg)
- **Reconstitution:** Not specified
- **Compatible Solutions:** Not specified

■ **IV Push:** Yes; may give undiluted
■ **IV Push Rate:** 10 mg slowly over 3–5 minutes
■ **IVPB:** No
■ **Special Considerations:** Administering concurrently with nonopioid analgesics may have additive effects and permit lower opioid doses

Naloxone (Narcan)

■ **Common Adult Dose:** 0.02–0.2 mg q 2–3 minutes until response obtained; repeat q 1–2 hours if needed
■ **Common Child Dose:** 5–10 mcg q 2–3 minutes repeated until response obtained; repeat q 1–2 hours if needed
■ **Solution Amount:** For infusion mix 2 mg in 500 ml for a final concentration of 4 mcg/ml
■ **Compatible Solutions:** D$_5$W, 0.9% NaCl,
■ **IV Push:** Yes; undiluted
■ **IV Push Rate:** 0.1–0.4 mg over 15 seconds
■ **IVPB:** Yes
■ **IV Infusion Time:** As a continuous infusion—titrate to the desired effect using an infusion pump
■ **Special Considerations:** Infusion solutions are stable for 24 hours

Neostigmine (Prostigmin)

■ **Common Adult Dose:** 0.5–2 mg slowly—pretreat with atropine 0.6–1.2 mg
■ **Common Child Dose:** 40 mcg/kg with 20 µg/kg atropine
■ **Reconstitution:** Not specified
■ **Compatible Solutions:** D$_5$W, 0.9% NaCl, Ringer's solution, LR
■ **IV Push:** Yes; administer doses undiluted
■ **IV Push Rate:** Each 0.5 mg over 1 minute through Y-site of a compatible solution
■ **IVPB:** No
■ **Special Considerations:** The pretreatment with atropine is used to prevent bradycardia

Nesiritide (Natrecor)

- **Common Adult Dose:** 2 mcg/kg bolus followed by 0.01 μg/kg/min as a continuous infusion
- **Reconstitution:** Remove 5 ml from a prefilled 250 ml plastic IV bag of a preservative-free compatible solution and add to vial; do not shake vial; rock gently so all surfaces including stopper are in contact with diluent to ensure complete reconstitution; withdraw entire contents of vial and add to a 250 ml plastic IV bag for a concentration of 6 mcg/ml—invert bag several times to mix
  - Prime tubing with an infusion of 25 ml before connecting to patient's vascular access port and before a bolus or infusion
  - Flush line between administration of nesiritide and other medications
  - Do not administer through a central heparin-coated catheter: it binds to heparin; can administer heparin through a separate IV line
- **Compatible Solutions:** D_5W, 0.9% NaCl, D5/0.45% NaCl, D5/0.2% NaCl
- **IV Push:** Yes: after preparing infusion bag, withdraw bolus amount from bag; calculate amount—bolus volume = 0.33 × patient weight (kg); do not use a higher dose than recommended 2 mcg/kg dose
- **IV Push Rate:** Administer bolus over 60 seconds through Y-site of a compatible solution
- **IVPB:** Yes: after bolus, immediately administer infusion; calculate infusion—infusion flow rate (ml/hr = 0.1 × patient weight [kg]); do not increase dose more frequently than q 3 hours to a maximum dose of 0.3 mcg/kg/min
- **Special Considerations:** Administer only in settings where BP is consistently monitored

Netilmicin (Netromycin)

- **Common Adult Dose:** 1.3–2.2 q 8 hours or 2–3.25 mg/kg q 12 hours
- **Common Child Dose:** 1.83–3.25 mg/kg every 12 hours
- **Reconstitution:** N/A
- **Solution Amount:** 50–200 ml (dilute in smaller proportionate volume for children)
- **Compatible Solutions:** D5/LR, D5/0.9% NaCl D_5W, $D_{10}W$, Ringer's solution, LR, 0.9% NaCl, 3% NaCl, 5% NaCl
- **IV Push:** No
- **IVPB:** Yes
- **Infusion Time:** 30 minutes to 2 hours
- **Special Considerations:** Solutions may be pale yellow and still maintain potency

Nicardipine (Cardene IV)

- **Common Adult Dose:** *To replace PO use:* 0.5–2.2 mg/hr continuous infusion; *treat acute hypertensive episodes:* 5 mg/hr titrated as needed up to 15 mg/hr
- **Reconstitution:** Not specified
- **Compatible Solutions:** D_5W, D5/0.45% NaCl, D5/0.9% NaCl, D5/KCl 40 mEq, 0.45% NaCl, 0.9% NaCl
- **IV Push:** No
- **IVPB:** No
- **Continuous Infusion:** Yes; dilute each 25 mg ampule with 240 ml of a compatible solution to a concentration of 0.1 mg/ml
- **Infusion Time:** Administer slowly and titrate rate according to BP response
- **Special Considerations:** Continuous infusions of 0.5 mg/hr, 1.2 mg/hr, and 2.2 mg/hr produce average plasma concentrations equal to a 20 mg, 30 mg, and 40 mg oral dose

Nitroglycerin (Tridil)

- **Common Adult Dose:** 5 mcg/min; can increase by 5 mcg/min q 3–5 minutes to 20 mcg/min, then increase by 10–20 mcg/min q 3–5 minutes (dosing determined by hemodynamic parameters)
- **Reconstitution:** Not specified
- **Compatible Solutions:** D₅W, 0.9% NaCl
- **IV Push:** No
- **IVPB:** No
- **IV Continuous Infusion:** Yes: doses must be diluted and administered as an infusion; use glass bottles only and special tubing provided by the manufacturer; dilute in a compatible solution for a concentration of 25–40 mcg/ml
- **Infusion Time:** Administer via infusion pump to ensure accurate rate; titrate rate according to patient's response
- **Special Considerations:** Nitroglycerine should not be admixed with other medications

Nitroprusside (Nitropress)

- **Common Adult and Child Dose:** 0.3 mcg/kg/min initially—may be increased as needed up to 10 mcg/kg/min—usual dose of 3 mcg/kg/min, not to exceed 10 minutes of therapy at 10 mcg/kg/min infusion rate
- **Reconstitution:** Reconstitute each 50 mg with 2–3 ml of D₅W for preservative-free injection
- **Compatible Solutions:** D₅W; do not admix with other medications
- **IV Push:** No
- **IVPB:** Yes: after reconstitution, dilute further in 250–1000 ml D₅W for a concentration of 200–500 mcg/ml; wrap infusion bottle in aluminum foil to protect from light—tubing need not be covered
- **Infusion Time:** Administer via infusion pump for accurate dosage rate
- **Special Considerations:** Fresh-prepared solution is slightly brownish; discard if dark brown, orange, blue, green, or dark red
- Requires cardiac monitoring and continuous BP monitoring

Octreotide (Sandostatin, Sandostatin LAR)

- **Common Adult Dose:** *Antidiarrheal:* 100–1800 mcg/day (unlabeled); *carcinoid tumors—Sandostatin:* 100–600 mcg/day in 2–4 divided doses during first 2 weeks of therapy
- **Compatible Solutions:** 0.9% NaCl, D₅W
- **Solution Amount:** Dilute in 50–200 ml of a compatible solution
- **IV Push:** Bolus used in emergency situations
- **IVPB:** Yes; dilute in 50–200 ml of a compatible solution
- **Infusion Time:** Administer over 15–30 minutes
- **Special Considerations:** Assess frequency and consistency of stools and bowel sounds during therapy

Ofloxacin (Floxin)

- **Common Adult Dose:** 200–400 mg q 12 hours
- **Common Child Dose:** N/A
- **Reconstitution:** Dilute to a concentration of 4 mg/ml
- **Solution Amount:** Dilute to a concentration of 4 mg/ml
- **Compatible Solutions:** D₅W, 0.9% NaCl, 0.9% NaCl, D5/LR, 5% sodium bicarbonate, D5, Plasmalyte 56, sodium lactate
- **IV Push:** No
- **IVPB:** Yes
- **IV Infusion Time:** 60 minutes
- **Special Considerations:** Discard unused portions

Ondansetron (Zofran)

- **Common Adult Dose:** 0.15 mg/kg 15–30 minutes prechemotherapy; repeat 4 and 8 hours later, or 32 mg single dose 30 minutes prechemotherapy
- **Common Child Dose:** 0.15 mg/kg 15–30 minutes prechemotherapy; repeat 4 and 8 hours later
- **Reconstitution:** Not specified
- **Solution Amount:** 50 ml
- **Compatible Solutions:** D₅W, 0.9% NaCl, D5/0.9% NaCl, D5/0.45% NaCl

- **IV Push:** Yes
- **IV Push Rate:** Over at least 30 seconds, but preferably over 2–5 minutes
- **IVPB:** Yes
- **Infusion Time:** Over 15 minutes
- **Special Considerations:** Do not confuse with **Zosyn**

Orphenadrine (Flexon, Norflex)

- **Common Adult Dose:** 60 mg q 12 hours
- **Reconstitution:** Not specified
- **Compatible Solutions:** Not specified
- **IV Push:** Yes: may be administered undiluted
- **Special Considerations:** Do not confuse with **Norfloxacin**

Oxymorphone (Numorphan)

- **Common Adult Dose:** 0.5 mg q 3–6 hours prn; increase as needed
- **Reconstitution:** Not specified
- **Compatible Solutions:** Not specified
- **IV Push:** Yes
- **IV Push Rate:** Undiluted over 2–3 minutes
- **IVPB:** No
- **Special Considerations:** Accidental overdose of opioid analgesics has resulted in death; clarify all orders with a practitioner before administering

Oxytocin (Pitocin)

- **Common Adult Dose:** 0.5–2 mU/min to induce labor, then increasing by 1–2 mU q 15–60 minutes; for hemorrhage—10 units
- **Reconstitution:** N/A
- **Solution Amount:** 1 ml (10 units) in 1 liter of solution

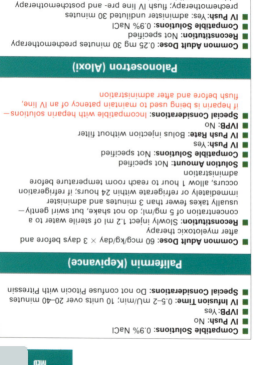

- **Compatible Solutions:** 0.9% NaCl
- **IV Push:** No
- **IVPB:** Yes
- **IV Infusion Time:** 0.5–2 mU/min; 10 units over 20–40 minutes
- **Special Considerations:** Do not confuse Pitocin with Pitressin

Palifermin (Kepivance)

- **Common Adult Dose:** 60 mcg/kg/day × 3 days before and after myelotoxic therapy
- **Reconstitution:** Slowly inject 1.2 ml of sterile water to a concentration of 5 mg/ml; do not shake, but swirl gently— usually takes fewer than 3 minutes and administer immediately or refrigerate within 24 hours; if refrigeration occurs, allow 1 hour to reach room temperature before administration
- **Solution Amount:** Not specified
- **Compatible Solutions:** Not specified
- **IV Push:** Yes
- **IV Push Rate:** Bolus injection without filter
- **IVPB:** No
- **Special Considerations:** Incompatible with heparin solutions— if heparin is being used to maintain patency of an IV line, flush before and after administration

Palonosetron (Aloxi)

- **Common Adult Dose:** 0.25 mg 30 minutes prechemotherapy
- **Reconstitution:** Not specified
- **Compatible Solutions:** 0.9% NaCl
- **IV Push:** Yes: administer undiluted 30 minutes prechemotherapy; flush IV line pre- and postchemotherapy with a compatible solution
- **IVPB:** No
- **Special Considerations:** Do not mix with other drugs

Pamidronate (Aredia)

- **Common Adult Dose:** *Hypercalcemia of malignancy:* 30–90 mg; may be repeated in 7 days
- **Reconstitution:** Reconstitute with 10 ml sterile water to each vial for a concentration of 30 mg/10 ml, 60 mg/ml, 90 mg/ml; dissolve drug before withdrawing
- **Solution Amount:** 1000 ml
- **Compatible Solutions:** 0.45% NaCl, 0.9% NaCl, D_5W
- **IV Push:** No
- **IVPB:** Yes
- **Infusion Time:** 60 mg over at least 4 hours; 90 mg over 24 hours
- **Special Considerations:** Patients with severe hypercalcemia should be started with a 90 mg dose

Pantoprazole (Protonix)

- **Common Adult Dose:** 40–80 mg q 12–24 hours (up to 240 mg/day)
- **Common Child Dose:** N/A
- **Reconstitution:** 10 ml of 0.9% NaCl
- **Solution Amount:** 100 ml
- **Compatible Solutions:** D_5W, 0.9% NaCl, LR
- **IV Push:** Yes
- **IV Push Rate:** Reconstituted in 10 ml of 0.9% NaCl over 2 minutes
- **IVPB:** Yes
- **IV Infusion Time:** 15 minutes
- **Special Considerations:** Administer through the filter provided to remove precipitates that may form when solution is mixed

Penicillins (Pencillinase-Resistant Nafcillin)

- **Common Adult Dose:** 500–1500 mg/kg q 12 hours
- **Common Child (and Infant) Dose:** 6.25–12.5 mg/kg q 6 hours

- **Reconstitution:** Add 3.4 ml of sterile water to each 1 g vial, or 6.8 ml sterile water to each 2 g vial for a concentration of 250 mg/ml
- **Compatible Solutions:** 0.9% NaCl, D₅W, D₁₀W, D5/0.25% NaCl, D5/0.45% NaCl, D5/0.9% NaCl, D5/LR, Ringer's, LR
- **IV Push:** Yes
- **IV Push Rate:** Over 5–10 minutes
- **IVPB:** Yes: dilute to a concentration of 2–40 mg/ml with a compatible solution
- **Infusion Time:** Over at least 30–60 minutes
- **Special Considerations:** Assess vein for irritation and phlebitis

Penicillins (Penicillinase-Resistant Oxacillin)

- **Common Adult and Child ≥40 kg dose:** 250–2000 mg q 4–6 hours (no more than 20 g/day)
- **Common Child ≤40 kg dose:** 12.5–25 mg/kg q 6 hours or 16.7 mg/kg q 4 hours
- **Reconstitution:** Add 1.4 ml sterile water to 250 mg vial, 2.7 ml to each 500 mg vial, 5.7 ml to each 1 g vial, 11.5 ml to each 2 g vial, and 23 ml to each 4 g vial for a concentration of 250 mg/1.5 ml
- **Compatible Solutions:** 0.9% NaCl, D₅W, D5/0.9% NaCl, LR
- **IV Push:** Yes: further dilute each reconstituted 250 mg or 500 mg vial with 5 ml of sterile water or 0.9% NaCl, 10 ml for a 1 g vial, 20 ml for a 2 g vial, and 40 ml for a 4 g vial
- **IV Push Rate:** 10 minutes slowly
- **IVPB:** Yes: dilute to a concentration of 0.5–40 mg/ml with a compatible solution
- **Infusion Time:** Infuse for up to 6 hours
- **Special Considerations:** Assess vein for irritation and phlebitis
  - Administer immediately after reconstitution or within 4 hours if refrigerated
  - Do not filter administration
  - Do not mix with other diluents or medications
  - Discard unused medication 4 hours after reconstitution

Penicillins (Penicillin G)

- **Common Adult Dose:** 1–5 million units q 4–6 hours
- **Common Child Dose:** 8333–16,667 units/kg q 4 hours, 12,550–25,000 units/kg q 6 hours; up to 250,000–300,000 units/kg/day in divided doses
- **Reconstitution:** Reconstitute according to manufacturer's instructions—with sterile water for injection, D_5W, 0.9% NaCl
- **Compatible Solutions:** D_5W, 0.9% NaCl
- **IV Push:** No
- **IVPB:** Yes: 3 million or fewer doses should be diluted in at least 50 ml of a compatible solution; 3 million or more doses should be diluted in at least 100 ml of a compatible solution
- **Infusion Time:** Infuse over 1–2 hours in adults and 15–30 minutes in children
- **Continuous Infusion:** Yes: 10 million units or more doses may be diluted in 1 or 2 l and infused over 24 hours
- **Special Considerations:** Do not confuse with **Penicillin G Procaine**

Pentamidine (NebuPent, Pentam 300)

- **Common Adult and Child Dose:** 4 mg/kg once daily for 14–21 days
- **Reconstitution:** Add 3–5 ml of sterile water or D_5W to a 300 mg vial for a concentration of 100, 75, or 60 mg/ml
- **Compatible Solutions:** D_5W
- **IV Push:** No
- **IVPB:** Yes: dilute further in 50–250 ml of D_5W
- **Infusion Time:** Administer over 1–2 hours slowly
- **Special Considerations:** Educate patient to notify physician if fever, sore throat, signs of infection, bleeding gums, bloody stools, blood in urine, bruising, or petechiae occur

Phenobarbital (Luminal)

- **Common Adult Dose:** *Anticonvulsant:* 100–320 mg as needed initially—total of 600 mg in 24 hours
- **Common Child Dose:** *Anticonvulsant:* 10–20 mg/kg initially, then 1–6 mg/kg/day
- **Reconstitution:** Add a minimum of 3 ml of sterile water to sterile powder—further dilute with 10 ml of sterile water—if not absolutely clear within 5 minutes, do not use
- **Compatible Solutions:** Not specified
- **IV Push:** Yes
- **IV Push Rate:** Administer each 60 mg over at least 1 minute
- **IVPB:** No
- **Special Considerations:** Rapid administration may result in respiratory depression; keep 5% procaine solution available for extravasation; apply moist heat if extravasation occurs

Phentolamine (Regitine)

- **Common Adult Dose:** 5 mg 1–2 hours preoperative and repeated as necessary; add 10 mg to every 1000 ml of fluid containing norepinephrine
- **Common Child Dose:** 1 mg or 0.1 mg/kg given 1–2 hours preoperative repeated as necessary
- **Reconstitution:** Reconstitute each 5 mg with 1 ml of sterile water for injection or 0.9% NaCl; discard unused portion
- **Solution Amount:** 500 ml
- **Compatible Solutions:** D_5W
- **IV Push:** Yes
- **IV Push Rate:** 5 mg over 1 minute
- **IVPB:** Yes, added to infusions of vasoactive drips
- **IV Infusion Time:** 0.5–1 mg/min during surgery; titrate infusion according to patient response
- **Special Considerations:** Will not affect the pressor effect when added to these agents in drips; will prevent dermal necrosis possible with vasoconstrictive agents

Phenytoin (Dilantin)

- **Common Adult Dose:** *Anticonvulsant:* 15–20 mg/kg (loading); 100 mg q 6–8 hours (maintenance); *Antidysrhythmic:* 50–100 mg q 10–15 minutes until dysrhythmia abolished, or until 15 mg/kg has been administered, or until toxicity occurs
- **Common Child Dose:** 15–20 mg/kg
- **Reconstitution:** N/A
- **Solution Amount:** 50 ml or mix to a concentration of 1–10 mg/ml
- **Compatible Solutions:** 0.9% NaCl only
- **IV Push:** Yes
- **IVPB:** Yes
- **IV Push Rate:** Do not exceed 50 mg/min or hypotension may occur
- **IV Infusion Time:** 1 hour; do not exceed an infusion rate of 50 mg/min
- **Special Considerations:** Do not refrigerate—precipitate may form
  - Must be administered into 0.9% NaCl solution
  - Flush line before and after administration with 0.9% NaCl if there are medications in the line

Phytonadione (Aquamephyton)

- **Common Adult Dose:** 2.5–10 mg; repeat in 12–48 hours if necessary
- **Common Child Dose:** *Infants:* 1–2 mg; *Children:* 2–5 mg
- **Reconstitution:** N/A
- **Solution Amount:** May be diluted in any amount if desired
- **Compatible Solutions:** D_5W, D5/0.9% NaCl, 0.9% NaCl
- **IV Push:** Yes
- **IV Push Rate:** Very slowly—do not exceed 1 mg/min
- **IVPB:** Yes
- **IV Infusion Time:** Very slowly—do not exceed 1 mg/min
- **Special Considerations:** Use of IV phytonadione should be reserved for emergencies

Piperacillin (Pipracil)

- **Common Adult Dose:** 3–4 g q 6–12 hours
- **Common Child Dose:** 50 mg/kg q 6–12 hours
- **Reconstitution:** Reconstitute with 5 ml of 0.9% NaCl, sterile or bacteriostatic water for injection, or D₅W; do not use LR; shake well until dissolved
- **Solution Amount:** 50 ml
- **Compatible Solutions:** D₅W, 0.9% NaCl
- **IV Push:** No
- **IVPB:** Yes
- **IV Infusion Time:** At least 30 minutes
- **Special Considerations:** Stable for 24 hours at room temperature and 48 hours if refrigerated

Piperacillin/Tazobactam (Zosyn)

- **Common Adult Dose:** 3.375–4.5 g q 6 hours
- **Common Child Dose:** N/A
- **Reconstitution:** Reconstitute with 5 ml of 0.9% NaCl, sterile or bacteriostatic water for injection, or D₅W; do not use LR; shake well until dissolved
- **Solution Amount:** 50 ml
- **Compatible Solutions:** D₅W, 0.9% NaCl, D5/0.9% NaCl, LR
- **IV Push:** Yes
- **IV Push Rate:** Slowly over 3–5 minutes
- **IVPB:** Yes
- **IV Infusion Time:** At least 20–30 minutes for adults, 30 minutes for children
- **Special Considerations:** Stable for 24 hours at room temperature and 48 hours if refrigerated

Potassium Acetate, Potassium Chloride

- **Common Adult Dose:** Up to 200 mEq/day as an infusion
- **Common Child Dose:** Up to 3 mEq/kg/day as an infusion
- **Reconstitution:** N/A
- **Solution Amount:** 100–1000 ml
- **Compatible Solutions:** D_5W, $D_{10}W$, D5/0.25% NaCl, D5/0.45% NaCl, D5/0.9% NaCl, 0.9% NaCl, LR, D5/LR
- **IV Push:** NEVER!
- **IVPB:** Yes: as an infusion
- **IV Infusion Time:** Infuse at a rate of 10 mEq/hr
- **Special Considerations:** Limited to 40 mEq/l infused into a peripheral line; up to 100 mEq/l via a central line

Potassium Phosphate

- **Common Adult Dose:** 10 mmol phosphorus/day
- **Common Child Dose:** (infants) 1.5–2 mmol phosphorus/day
- **Reconstitution:** Not specified
- **Solution Amount:** Administer only in dilute concentrations of no greater than 160 mEq/ml with a compatible solution
- **Compatible Solutions:** D_5W, $D_{10}W$, D5/0.45% NaCl, D5/0.9% NaCl, 0.9% NaCl, 0.45% NaCl, TPN solutions
- **IV Push:** No
- **IVPB:** No
- **Continuous Infusion:** Yes
- **Continuous Infusion Rate:** Maximum dose over 24 hours—not to exceed 0.24 mmol/kg/day—give over 6 hours
- **Special Considerations:** Do not administer undiluted; may cause precipitate in solutions containing calcium; do not mix with other medications

Prednisolone (Delta-Cortef)

- **Common Adult Dose:** 4–60 mg/day
- **Common Child Dose:** 0.14 mg/kg/day in 3 divided doses
- **Reconstitution:** May be administered undiluted
- **Solution Amount:** 50–1000 ml as an intermittent infusion or as a continuous infusion
- **Compatible Solutions:** D_5W, 0.9% NaCl
- **IV Push:** Yes
- **IV Push Rate:** 10 mg/min
- **IV Infusion Time:** Not specified
- **Special Considerations:** Do not use the acetate form for IV administration

Procainamide (Pronestyl)

- **Common Adult Dose:** 100 mg q 5 minutes until dysrhythmia is abolished, or 100 mg has been given, or loading dose infusion of 500–600 mg followed by a maintenance infusion of 2–6 mg/min
- **Common Child Dose:** N/A
- **Reconstitution:** Dilute each 100 mg with 10 ml of D_5W or sterile water for injection
- **Solution Amount:** Add 200 mg to 1 g to 50–500 ml, for a concentration of 2–4 mg/ml
- **Compatible Solutions:** D_5W
- **IV Push:** Yes
- **IV Push Rate:** 25–50 mg/min—rapid administration may cause ventricular fibrillation or asystole
- **IVPB:** Yes
- **IV Infusion Time:** Loading dose—30 minutes; maintenance infusion: 2–6 mg/min
- **Special Considerations:** Solution is slightly yellow in color; do not use if solution is darker than light amber or if contains precipitate
- Requires cardiac monitoring

Prochlorperazine (Compazine)

- **Common Adult Dose:** *Antiemetic:* 2.5–10 mg (not to exceed 40 mg) may be repeated once; *Antipsychotic:* 2.5–10 mg (not to exceed 40 mg); *Antianxiety:* 2.5–10 mg (not to exceed 40 mg)
- **Common Child Dose:** Give only to children over 12 years; dose is the same as adult dose
- **Reconstitution:** Dilute to a concentration of 1 mg/ml; can dilute 20 mg in up to 1 liter
- **Solution Amount:** Up to 1 liter
- **Compatible Solutions:** D_5W, $D_{10}W$, D5/0.25% NaCl, D5/0.45% NaCl, D5/0.9% NaCl, 0.9% NaCl, LR, D5/LR, Ringer's
- **IV Push:** Yes
- **IV Push Rate:** 1 mg/min, not to exceed 5 mg/min
- **IVPB:** Yes
- **IV Infusion Time:** Not specified, but infusion time should not exceed 5 mg/min
- **Special Considerations:** Do not confuse with **chlorpromazine**

Promethazine (Phenergan)

- **Common Adult Dose:** 10–25 mg q 4 hours
- **Common Child Dose:** N/A
- **Reconstitution:** N/A
- **Compatible Solutions:** D_5W, $D_{10}W$, D5/0.25% NaCl, D5/0.45% NaCl, D5/0.9% NaCl, 0.9% NaCl, LR, D5/LR
- **IV Push:** Yes
- **IV Push Rate:** 25 mg over 1 minute
- **IVPB:** No
- **Special Considerations:** Rapid injection may cause a drop in BP
  - Slight yellow color does not alter potency
  - Do not use if precipitate present

Propranolol (Inderal)

- **Common Adult Dose:** 1–3 mg may be repeated after 2 minutes and again in 4 hours if needed
- **Common Child Dose:** 10–100 mcg (0.01–0.1 mg/kg [up to 1 mg/dose]); may be repeated q 6–8 hours if needed
- **Reconstitution:** May be administered undiluted or may dilute each 1 mg in 10 ml of D₅W for injection
- **Solution Amount:** 50 ml
- **Compatible Solutions:** D₅W, D5/0.45% NaCl, D5/0.9% NaCl, 0.9% NaCl, LR
- **IV Push:** Yes
- **IV Push Rate:** Over at least 1 minute
- **IVPB:** Yes
- **IV Infusion Time:** 10–15 minutes
- **Special Considerations:** Oral and parenteral dose of propranolol are not interchangeable; the IV dose is 1/10 the oral dose

Protamine Sulfate

- **Common Adult and Child Dose:** *heparin overdosage:* 1 mg/100 units of heparin; if <30 minutes, give 0.5 mg/100 units of heparin; not to exceed 100 mg/2 hr; *Enoxaparin overdosage:* 1 mg/each mg of enoxaparin; *Dalteparin overdosage:* 1 mg/100 anti-Xa IU of dalteparin; if required, a second dose of 0.5 mg/100 anti-Xa IU of dalteparin may be given 2–4 hours later if laboratory studies indicate a need
- **Reconstitution:** Reconstitute 50 mg vial with 5 ml and 250 mg vial with 25 ml of sterile water for injection or bacteriostatic water for injection for a concentration of 10 mg/ml; shake vigorously
- **Solution Amount:** Not specified
- **Compatible Solutions:** D₅W, 0.9% NaCl
- **IV Push:** Yes
- **IV Push Rate:** May be administered undiluted over 1–3 minutes

- **IVPB:** Yes
- **IV Infusion Time:** 50 mg over 10 minutes
- **Special Considerations:** Solution reconstituted with sterile water should be discarded after dose is withdrawn; solutions reconstituted with bacteriostatic water are stable for 24 hours when refrigerated
  - Rapid infusion may result in hypotension, bradycardia, flushing, or feeling of warmth; if these symptoms occur, stop infusion and notify physician

Pyridostigmine (Mestinon)

- **Common Adult Dose:** *Myasthenia gravis:* 2 mg; may be repeated q 2–3 hours; *Antidote for nondepolarizing neuromuscular blockade:* 10–20 mg (pretreat with 0.6–1.2 mg atropine IV)
- **Common Child Dose:** N/A
- **Recompatible Solutions:** D₅W, 0.9% NaCl, LR, D5/LR, D5/Ringer's solution
- **IV Push:** Yes; may be administered undiluted
- **IV Push Rate:** Myasthenia gravis: 0.5 mg over 1 minute; reversal of nondepolarizing neuromuscular blocking agent: 5 mg over 1 minute
- **IVPB:** No

Pyridoxine (Beesix)

- **Common Adult Dose:** *Pyridoxine–dependency syndrome:* 30–600 mg/day; *Isoniazid overdose:* amount in milligrams equal to amount of isoniazid ingested, given as 4 g IV, then an IM dose
- **Common Child Dose:** *Pyridoxine-dependency syndrome:* 30–600 mg/day
- **Solution Amount:** Not specified; may be administered undiluted direct IV or as an infusion
- **Compatible Solutions:** Standard IV solutions
- **IV Push:** Yes
- **IV Push Rate:** 15–30 minutes
- **IVPB:** Yes
- **IV Infusion Time:** Up to 3 hours

Quinidine Gluconate (Quiniglute)

- **Common Adult Dose:** 16 mg/min until dysrhythmia is suppressed, QRS complex widens, bradycardia or hypotension occurs
- **Common Child Dose:** N/A
- **Reconstitution:** N/A
- **Solution Amount:** Dilute 800 mg (10 ml) in 50 ml (concentration of 16 mg/ml)
- **Compatible Solutions:** D₅W
- **IV Push:** No
- **IVPB:** Yes
- **IV Infusion Time:** Administer via infusion pump at a rate not to exceed 1 ml/min
- **Special Considerations:** Stable for 24 hours at room temperature and 48 hours if refrigerated
- Rapid administration may cause peripheral vascular collapse and severe hypotension
- Use only clear colorless solutions

Quinupristin/Dalfopristin (Synercid)

- **Common Adult Dose:** 7.5 mg/kg q 8–12 hours for at least 7 days
- **Common Child Dose:** N/A
- **Reconstitution:** Reconstitute by slowly adding 5 ml of D₅W or sterile water for injection for a concentration of 100 mg/ml; gently swirl to mix; avoid shaking to prevent foam formation; allow solution to sit until all foam has disappeared
- **Solution Amount:** 250 ml (100 ml for central line infusion)
- **Compatible Solutions:** D₅W
- **IV Push:** No
- **IVPB:** Yes
- **IV Infusion Time:** Over 60 minutes using an infusion pump
- **Special Considerations:** Solution should be clear
- Solution is stable at room temperature for 5 hours and 54 hours if refrigerated
- Flush line before and after infusion with D₅W
- Do not use 0.9% NaCl or heparin

Ranitidine (Zantac)

- **Common Adult Dose:** 50 mg q 6–8 hours (not to exceed 400 mg/day); may be given as a continuous infusion of 6.25 mg/hr
- **Common Child Dose:** N/A
- **Reconstitution:** N/A
- **Solution Amount:** 100 ml; continuous infusion—150 mg/250 ml of D_5W
- **Compatible Solutions:** D_5W, 0.9% NaCl
- **IV Push:** Yes; dilute each 50 mg in 20 ml of 0.9% NaCl or D_5W for injection
- **IVPB:** Yes
- **IV Push Rate:** Administer over at least 5 minutes
- **IV Infusion Time:** 15–30 minutes
- **Special Considerations:** Do not use solution that is discolored or that contains precipitate

Rasburicase (Elitek)

- **Common Adult Dose:** N/A
- **Common Child Dose:** 0.15 or 0.2 mg/kg single dose daily for 5 days; dose determined by patient's weight and dose/kg
- **Reconstitution:** Diluent provided; add 1 ml and swirl gently—do not shake
- **Solution Amount:** 50 ml of a compatible solution
- **Compatible Solutions:** 0.9% NaCl
- **IV Push:** No
- **IVPB:** Yes
- **IV Infusion Time:** 30 minutes' infusion
- **Special Considerations:** Do not administer as a bolus; infuse through separate IV line; do not use if solution discolored or particulate material is present

Reteplase (Retavase)

- **Common Adult Dose:** 10 U; repeat dose 30 minutes later
- **Reconstitution:** Diluent and equipment provided; do not shake; swirl vial to mix. If foaming occurs, let vial stand for a few minutes; administer immediately after mixing
- **Compatible Solutions:** D₅W
- **IV Push:** Yes
- **IV Push Rate:** Over 2 minutes into a D₅W IV line—flush line before and after
- **IVPB:** No
- **Special Considerations:** Incompatible with heparin; line should be used only for this drug; do not add other drugs to this IV line

Rh(D) Globulin IV (WinRho)

- **Common Adult Dose:** *Following delivery:* 600 IU within 72 hours of delivery. *Before delivery:* 1500 IU at 28 weeks; if before 28 weeks repeat q 12 weeks. *Following amniocentesis:* 1500 IU within 72 hours; repeat q 12 weeks during pregnancy. *Large fetal-maternal hemorrhage/Transfusion accident:* 3000 IU q 8 hours until dose completed; total dose determined by amount of blood loss; *Immune thrombocytopenic purpura (ITP):* 50 mcg/kg initially; 25–40 mcg if Hgb < 10 g/dl; further dosing determined by response (range 25–60 mcg/kg); may be given as a divided dose on separate days or as a singe dose
- **Common Child Dose:** *Immune thrombocytopenic purpura (ITP):* 50 mcg/kg initially; 25–40 mcg if Hgb < 10 g/dl; further dosing determined by response (range 25–60 mcg/kg); may be given as a divided dose on separate days or as a singe dose
- **Reconstitution:** Reconstitute immediately before use with 2.5 ml of 0.9% NaCl; inject diluent onto inside wall of vial, and wet pellet by gently swirling until dissolved; do not shake
- **IV Push:** Yes
- **IV Push Rate:** 3–5 minutes
- **IVPB:** No

Rifampin (Rifadin)

- **Common Adult Dose:** *Tuberculosis:* 10 mg/kg/day (up to 600 mg/day as a single dose or 2–3 times per week; *Asymptomatic carrier of meningococcus:* 600 mg q 12 hours for 2 days
- **Common Child Dose:** *Tuberculosis:* 10–20 mg/kg/day single dose (not to exceed 600 mg/day) may be given 2–3 times per week; *Asymptomatic carrier of meningococcus:* 10 mg/kg q 12 hours for 2 days
- **Reconstitution:** 10 ml of sterile water for injection, and swirl gently to dissolve completely
- **Solution Amount:** 100 or 500 ml
- **Compatible Solutions:** D_5W, 0.9% NaCl
- **IV Push:** No
- **IVPB:** Yes
- **IV Infusion Time:** 500 ml over 3 hours and 100 ml over 30 minutes
- **Special Considerations:** Administer within 4 hours to prevent precipitation; stable for 24 hours at room temperature

Sargramostim (Leukine)

- **Common Adult Dose:** Depending on medical problem—250 mcg/m² × 14 days; may repeat after a 7-day rest; if results are still inadequate, may give 500 mcg/m² × 14 days after a 7–day rest. *After bone-marrow transplantation*—250 mcg/m² × 21 days
- **Reconstitution:** Add 1 ml of sterile water (no preservatives) to vial by injecting the solution toward the side of the vial; do not shake, but swirl gently; the solution will be clear and colorless; single-dose vial only
- **Solution Amount:** Concentrations should be >1 mcg/ml; if not, add 1 mg/ml of albumin to 0.9% NaCl before adding the medication
- **Compatible Solutions:** 0.9% NaCl
- **IV Push:** No
- **IVPB:** Yes

- **IV Infusion Time:** 2–4 hours
- **Continuous Infusion:** Yes—over 24 hours
- **Special Considerations:** Refrigerate, but do not freeze powder; **Do not confuse with Leukeran**

Scopolamine

- **Common Adult Dose:** 0.2–0.6 mg 3–4 times daily
- **Common Child Dose:** 6 mcg/kg or 0.2 mg/m²
- **Solution Amount:** Dilute with 10 ml of a compatible solution before administration
- **Compatible Solutions:** Sterile water
- **IV Push:** Yes
- **IV Push Rate:** Inject slowly over 1 minute
- **IVPB:** No
- **Special Considerations:** Monitor heart rate; because scopolamine can act as a stimulant in the presence of pain, assess pain before administration

Sodium Bicarbonate

- **Common Adult and Child Dose:** *Urine alkalinization:* 2–5 mEq/kg; *Systemic alkalinization/Cardiac arrest:* 1 mEq/kg and may repeat 0.5 mEq/kg q 10 minutes
- **Solution Amount:** Dilute in a compatible solution
- **Compatible Solutions:** D₅W, 0.9% NaCl, dextrose/saline
- **IV Push:** Yes: in a cardiac arrest circumstance—base dose on ABG results, and may be repeated q 10 minutes
- **IV Push Rate:** May be given as rapid bolus
- **IVPB:** No
- **Continuous Infusion:** Yes
- **Infusion Time:** May be given over 4–8 hours
- **Special Consideration:**
- **HOT TIP!** Flush line before and after to prevent arrest management incompatible medications from precipitating

Sodium Chloride

- **Common Adult Dose**: *Rate and amount determined by condition being treated:* 0.9% NaCl (1 l), 0.45% NaCl (1–2 l); 3%–5% NaCl 100 ml/hr
- **Compatible Solutions**: D_5W, $D_{10}W$, D5/0.25% NaCl, D5/0.45% NaCl, D5/0.9% NaCl, 0.9% NaCl, LR, D5/LR
- **IVPB Infusion**: Yes—3% or 5% NaCl must be administered in a large vein, and avoid infiltration
- **IV Infusion Time**: Hypertonic NaCl solutions should not exceed 100 ml/hr
- **Special Considerations**: 0.9% NaCl—isotonic, 0.45% NaCl (hypotonic), 3% and 5% NaCl (hypertonic). Serious electrolyte imbalances have occurred with the accidental infusion of hypertonic NaCl solutions; do not confuse concentration NaCl with NaCl flush solutions

Sodium Ferric Gluconate Complex (Ferrlecit)

- **Common Adult Dose**: 10 ml (1.25 mg elemental iron) repeated during 8 sequential dialysis treatments for a cumulative dose of 1 g
- **Common Child Dose**: N/A
- **Reconstitution**: N/A
- **Solution Amount**: *Test dose:* 50 ml; *Therapeutic dose:* 100 ml
- **Compatible Solutions**: 0.9% NaCl
- **IV Push**: No
- **IVPB**: Yes
- **IV Infusion Time**: 2 ml (25 mg) should be administered as a test dose, diluted in 50 ml of 0.9% NaCl and administered over 60 minutes; therapeutic dose should be administered over 1 hour

Streptokinase (Streptase)

- **Common Adult Dose**: MI: 1.5 million IU; DVT, PE: 250,000 IU loading, then 100,000 IU/hr × 24 hours for PE and 72 hours for DVT; *Intracoronary*: 20,000 IU bolus, then 2000 IU/min infusion × 1 hour for a total dose of 140,000 IU
- **Reconstitution**: IVPB—Add 5 ml of a compatible solution to vial; swirl gently, do not shake
- **Solution Amount**: *Intracoronary*: Dilute the 250,000 IU vial for a total of 125 ml with a compatible solution. *IVPB or MI*: 45 ml; *DVT or PE*: 90 ml (increments to a total of up to 500 ml)
- **Compatible Solutions**: 0.9% NaCl, D_5W
- **IV Push**: Yes: *intracoronary*
- **IV Push Rate**: Give 20,000 IU (10 ml): 15 sec to 2 min bolus
- **IVPB**: Yes
- **IV Infusion Time**: *MI*: 1 hour; *Postintracoronary bolus*: infuse 2000 IU/min for 1 hour; *DVT or PE loading dose*: over 30 minutes, then an infusion of 100,000 IU/hr; *Cannula/Catheter clearance*: infused over 25–35 minutes into each occluded catheter lumen, then clamp for 2 hours; carefully withdraw contents and flush line with 0.9% NaCl
- **Special Considerations**: Solution may be slightly yellow in appearance; infusion pump must be used; may not be admixed with other medications

Tacrolimus (Prograf)

- **Common Adult Dose**: 0.05–0.1 mg/kg/day
- **Common Child Dose**: 0.1 mg/kg/day
- **Solution Amount**: Dilute with a compatible solution for a concentration of 0.004–0.02 mg/ml
- **Compatible Solutions**: 0.9% NaCl, D_5W
- **IV Push**: No
- **IVPB Infusion**: No
- **Continuous Infusion**: Yes
- **Infusion Rate**: Infuse over 24 hours
- **Special Considerations**: Observe for signs of anaphylaxis—if signs are noted, stop infusion and begin treatment

Tenecteplase (TNKase)

- **Common Adult Dose:** <60 kg = 30 mg; ≥60 kg and <70 kg = 35 mg; ≥70 kg and <80 kg = 40 mg; ≥80 kg and <90 kg = 45 mg; ≥90 kg = 50 mg
- **Reconstitution:** Items provided for dilution; use sterile water only, not bacteriostatic water; add 10 ml diluent to vial—inject directly into powder; if foaming occurs, let stand for a few minutes—do not shake; 5 mg/ml solution is pale yellow; see insert instructions for shield use
- **Compatible Solutions:** 0.9% NaCl
- **IV Push:** Yes
- **IV Push Rate:** Single bolus over 5 minutes
- **IVPB:** No
- **Special Considerations:** Not compatible with dextrose-containing solutions

Terbutaline

- **Common Adult Dose:** *Tocolysis:* During contractions, give 10 µg/min infusion and increase by 5 mcg/min q 10 minutes until contractions cease; once contractions have ceased for 30 minutes, decrease infusion rate until effectiveness maintained for 4–8 hours
- **Solution Amount:** Dilute in a compatible solution
- **Compatible Solutions:** D_5W, 0.9% NaCl, 0.45% NaCl
- **IV Push:** No
- **IVPB Infusion:** No
- **Continuous Infusion:** Yes
- **Infusion Time:** Begin at 10 mcg/min; dosage increased by 5 mcg/10 min until contractions cease—maximum dose 80 mcg/min; once contractions have ceased for 30–60 minutes, decrease dose in 5 mcg increments
- **Special Considerations:** Infusion pump must be used to ensure accurate dosage

Theophylline (Quibron T)

- **Common Adult and Child Dose (6 month to adult):** Loading Dose: 4.7 mg/kg, followed by an infusion of 0.55 mg/kg/hr for 12 hours, followed by 0.36 mg/kg/hr
- **Common Child Dose:** 1–3 mg/kg every 8–12 hours
- **Compatible Solutions:** D_5W
- **IV Push:** No
- **IV Infusion Time:** Loading dose should be infused over 20–30 minutes; longer infusions should not exceed 20–25 mg/min
- **Special Considerations:**
  - Must be infused on an infusion pump
  - Loading dose should be given in a small volume, and continuous infusion should be given in a larger volume

Thiamine (Biamine, Vitamin B1)

- **Common Adult Dose:** 5–100 mg tid
- **Common Child Dose:** 10–25 mg/day
- **Solution Amount:** Dilute in 1000 ml of a compatible solution
- **Compatible Solutions:** Dextrose/Ringer's or LR combinations, D_5W, $D_{10}W$, Ringer's, LR, 0.9% NaCl, 0.45% NaCl
- **IV Push:** Yes: undiluted
- **IV Push Rate:** Give at a rate of 100 mg over 5 minutes
- **IVPB:** No
- **Continuous Infusion:** Yes
- **Infusion Time:** Give over the ordered rate
- **Special Considerations:** Usually administered with other vitamins; incompatible with solutions with neutral or alkaline pH (carbonates, citrates, acetates)

Ticarcillin (Ticar)

- **Common Adult Dose:** 1–6 g in divided doses q 6 hours, depending on type of infection; not to exceed 24 g daily
- **Common Child Dose:** <40 kg to 12.5 mg to 75 mg/kg q 6 hours or q 8 hours depending on type of infection
- **Reconstitution:** Reconstitute with at least 4 ml of sterile water to each 1 g vial
- **Solution Amount:** 50–100 ml of a compatible solution
- **Compatible Solutions:** D_5W, 0.9% NaCl, Ringer's, LR
- **IV Push:** Yes: further dilute with 20 ml of a compatible solution
- **IV Push Rate:** Concentrations should not exceed 50 mg/ml—give as slowly as possible
- **IVPB:** Yes: dilute for a concentration of 10–100 mg/ml
- **IV Infusion Time:** Infuse over 30 minutes to 2 hours
- **Special Considerations:** If administering aminoglycosides and penicillins concurrently, must be given at least 1 hour apart in separate site

Ticarcillin/clavulanate (Timentin)

- **Common Adult Dose:** <60 kg to 33.3 mg to 75 mg/kg ticarcillin and 1.1–2.5 mg/kg clavulanate q 4–6 hours
- **Adults and Children:** ≥60 kg to 3.1 g q 4–6 hours
- **Common Child Dose:** ≥3 mo—<60 kg to 50–450 mg/kg ticarcillin and 1.7–17 mg/kg clavulanate q 4–6 hours in divided doses depending on medical problem
- **Reconstitution:** Add 13 ml of sterile water or 0.9% NaCl to each 3.1 g vial—ticarcillin concentration(200 mg/ml), clavulanate concentration (6.7 mg/ml)
- **Compatible Solutions:** D_5W, 0.9% NaCl, Ringer's, LR
- **IV Push:** Yes
- **IV Push Rate:** Over 30 minutes
- **IVPB:** Yes: Further dilute in a compatible solution
- **IV Infusion Time:** Over 30 minutes
- **Special Considerations:** If administering aminoglycosides and penicillins concurrently, must be given at least 1 hour apart in separate site

Tirofiban (Aggrastat)

- **Common Adult Dose**: 0.4 mcg/kg/min over 30 minutes
- **Common Child Dose**: N/A
- **Reconstitution**: N/A
- **Solution Amount**: N/A
- **Compatible Solutions**: Unavailable
- **IV Push**: Yes: administer undiluted for 2 minutes
- **IVPB**: No
- **IV Infusion Time**: N/A
- **Special Considerations**: Do not admix with other solutions or drugs

Tobramycin (Nebcin)

- **Common Adult Dose**: 0.75–1.25 mg/kg q 6 hours or 1–1.75 mg/kg q 8 hours
- **Reconstitution**: N/A
- **Solution Amount**: 50–100 ml
- **Compatible Solutions**: D_5W, $D_{10}W$, D5/0.9% NaCl, 0.9% NaCl, Ringer's solution, LR (maximum concentration 1 mg/ml)
- **IV Push**: No
- **IVPB**: Yes
- **IV Infusion Time**: 30–60 minutes

Torsemide (Demadex)

- **Common Adult Dose**: 5–20 mg once daily
- **Common Child Dose**: N/A
- **Reconstitution**: N/A
- **Solution Amount**: N/A
- **Compatible Solutions**: Not specified
- **IV Push**: Yes: administer undiluted for 2 minutes
- **IVPB**: No
- **IV Infusion Time**: N/A
- **Special Considerations**: Do not admix with other solutions or drugs

Trimethoprim (TMP)/Sulfamethoxazole (SMZ) (Bactrim, Septra)

- **Common Adult Dose:** 2–6.7 mg/kg TMP, 10–33.3 mg/kg SMZ q 6, 8, or 12 hours depending on the dose
- **Common Child Dose:** Same as adult dose for children >2 months
- **Reconstitution:** Each 5 ml ampule should be diluted with 100–125 ml of D_5W
- **Solution Amount:** 100–125 ml
- **Compatible Solutions:** D_5W, 0.9% NaCl
- **IV Push:** No
- **IVPB:** Yes
- **IV Infusion Time:** Infuse over 60–90 minutes; no bolus or rapid infusion
- **Special Considerations:** Do not refrigerate; do not admix with other medications or solutions

Urokinase (Abbokinase)

- **Common Adult Dose:** *For PE:* 4400 IU/kg loading dose, then 4400 IU/kg/hr × 12 hours
- **Reconstitution:** Add 5 ml sterile water (without preservatives) to 250,000 IU vial; swirl vial—do not shake; solution will be light straw–colored. Use immediately through a 0.45 micron filter
- **Solution Amount:** *For PE:* Dilute further with 190 ml 0.9% NaCl or D_5W
- **Compatible Solutions:** 0.9% NaCl, D_5W
- **IV Push:** No
- **IVPB:** Yes
- **IV Infusion Time:** *For PE:* loading dose over 10 minutes, then infusion of 4400 IU/kg/hr × 12 hours
- **Special Considerations:** Infusion pump must be used to ensure safe dose administration

Valproates (Depakote, Depacon, Depakene-Valproic Acid)

- **Common Adult Dose:** Initially 5–15 mg/kg/day, and increase by 5–10 mg/kg/day weekly until therapeutic levels are reached but not to exceed 60 mg/kg/day; if daily dose is over 250 mg, give in divided doses q 6 hours
- **Common Child Dose:** Same as adult dose in children > 10 years
- **Reconstitution:** N/A
- **Solution Amount:** 50 ml
- **Compatible Solutions:** D₅W, 0.9% NaCl, LR
- **IV Push:** No
- **IVPB:** Yes; dilute in a compatible solution
- **IV Infusion Time:** Infuse over 60 minutes not to exceed 20 mg/min
- **Special Considerations:** Infusions under 60 minutes can increase side effects of the drug

Vancomycin (Vancocin)

- **Common Adult Dose:** 500 mg q 6 hours to 1 g q 12 hours
- **Common Child Dose:** >1 month: 10 mg/kg q 6 hours or 20 mg/kg q 12 hours
- **Reconstitution:** Dilute 500 mg vial with 10 ml sterile water
- **Solution Amount:** Further dilute with 100–200 ml of a compatible solution
- **Compatible Solutions:** D₅W, 0.9% NaCl, D₁₀W, LR
- **IV Push:** No
- **IVPB:** Yes
- **IV Infusion Time:** Infuse over at least 1 hour
- **Special Considerations:** A 1–2 g/24 hours continuous infusion may be used if IVPB is not possible; never administer rapidly; rapid infusion can result in thrombophlebitis, hypotension, and "red person syndrome"

Vasopressin (Pitressin)

- **Common Adult Dose:** Single dose 40 units
- **Common Child Dose:** N/A
- **Solution Amount:** D_5W; dilute to a concentration of 0.1–1 U/ml
- **Compatible Solutions:** D_5W, 0.9% NaCl
- **IV Push:** Yes: Administer 40 units during cardiac arrest
- **IVPB:** No
- **Special Considerations:** Monitor ECG during therapy and consistently during CPR

Verapamil (Apo-Verap, Calan, Isoptin, Verelan)

- **Common Adult Dose:** (75–150 mcg/kg) 5–10 mg; can be repeated after 15–30 minutes with 10 mg (150 mcg/kg)
- **Common Child Dose:** *(1–15 years)* (100–300 mcg/kg) 2–5 mg (not to exceed 5 mg); can be repeated after 30 minutes, but not to exceed 10 mg); *(<1 yr):* (100–200 mcg/kg) 0.75–2 mg; can be repeated after 30 minutes
- **Solution Amount:** 5 ml of sterile water
- **Compatible Solutions:** Not specified
- **IV Push:** Yes: administer undiluted through Y-site over 2–3 minutes; in geriatric patients, administer over 3 minutes
- **IVPB:** No
- **Special Considerations:** To minimize a hypotensive occurrence, the patient should remain recumbent for at least 1 hour after medication IV administration
- Requires cardiac monitoring

Vitamin D compounds (Calcifediol, Doxercalciferol, Ergocalciferol, Paricalciol)

- **Common Adult Dose:** Calcitriol 0.5 mcg 3 times per week; dihydrotachysterol: 4 mcg 3 times per week; ergocalciferol as part of TPN, paricalciol 0.04–0.1 mcg/kg every other day
- **Common Child Dose:** As part of TPN
- **Reconstitution:** N/A
- **Solution Amount:** N/A
- **Compatible Solutions:** D$_5$W, D5/0.45 NaCl, D5/0.9% NaCl, 0.45% NaCl, 0.9% NaCl, D5/LR
- **IV Push:** Yes
- **IVPB:** Yes
- **IV Push Rate:** Calcitriol by rapid injection through the catheter at the end of a hemodialysis period
- **IV Infusion Rate:** As ordered by the physician

Voriconazole (VFEND)

- **Common Adult Dose:** Loading dose: 2 doses of 6 mg/kg q 12 hours, then maintenance dosing: 4 mg/kg q 12 hours
- **Common Child Dose:** Only to children >12 yr and > than 40 kg—2 doses of 6 mg/kg q 12 hours, then maintenance dosing: 4 mg/kg q 12 hours
- **Reconstitution:** Add 19 ml of sterile water to vial = 10 mg/ml concentration
- **Solution Amount:** Further dilute in a compatible solution for a dose concentration of 10 mg/ml by withdrawing and disposing of = diluent volume from the infusion bag; after adding the drug to the infusion bag, the concentration should not be <0.5 mg/ml or >5 mg/ml
- **Compatible Solutions:** D$_5$W, D5/20 mEq KCl, D5/0.9% NaCl, D5/LR, D5/0.45% NaCl, 0.9% NaCl, 0.45% NaCl, LR
- **IV Push:** No
- **IVPB:** Yes
- **IV Infusion Time:** Over 1–2 hours; do not exceed 3 mg/kg/hr
- **Special Considerations:** Infuse through a separate line; monitor liver function before and during therapy

Warfarin (Coumadin, Warfilone)

- **Common Adult Dose:** 2.5–10 mg/day for 2–4 days (see special considerations)
- **Common Child Dose:** N/A
- **Reconstitution:** Add 2.7 ml of sterile water to the vial
- **Compatible Solutions:** D_5W, D5/0.45% NaCl, D5/0.9% NaCl, 0.45% NaCl, 0.9% NaCl, D5/LR
- **IV Push:** Yes: administer slower over 1–2 minutes in a peripheral vein
- **IVPB:** No
- **Special Considerations:** Alter daily doses according to prothrombin time or INR results; the antidote is vitamin K for overdose effects

Zn-DTPA (Pentetate Zinc Trisodium)

- **Common Adult Dose: 12 years and older:** Length of treatment depends on extent and response to contamination. 1 g/day after Ca-DTPA
- **Common Child Dose:** <12 years: Length of treatment depends on extent and response to contamination. 14 mg/kg/day after Ca-DTPA
- **Reconstitution:** Not specified
- **Solution Amount:** 100–250 ml in a compatible solution
- **Compatible Solutions:** D_5W, 0.9% NaCl, LR
- **IV Push:** Yes
- **IV Push Rate:** Give undiluted over 3–4 minutes
- **IVPB:** Yes
- **IV Infusion Time:** Slow infusion
- **Special Considerations:** Give mineral or vitamin supplements as needed; patient should drink plenty of fluids and void frequently to dilute urine and prevent radiation damage to bladder; instruct patient to flush toilet several times after use

Zoledronic Acid (Zometa)

- **Common Adult Dose:** 4 mg q 3–4 weeks, but can be repeated after 7 days
- **Common Child Dose:** N/A
- **Reconstitution:** Add 5 ml of sterile water to each 4 mg vial
- **Solution Amount:** Further dilute with 100 ml of a compatible solution
- **Compatible Solutions:** D₅W, 0.9% NaCl
- **IV Push:** No
- **IVPB:** Yes
- **IV Infusion Time:** No more than 4 mg over at least 15 minutes in a separate IV line
- **Special Considerations:** Renal insufficiency and renal failure may occur with rapid infusion; do not mix with lactated Ringer's solution as it contains calcium

Critical Guidelines for Administration of Potassium

- **NEVER give potassium IV push (FATAL).**
- Do not give more than 120 mEq/24 hours without ICU monitoring.
- Potassium chloride (KCl) is compatible with most IV solutions.
- Never administer concentrated potassium without first diluting.
- Potassium solutions in commonly used strengths (20 or 40 mEq/L) are available in premixed form from manufacturers.
- KCl preparations greater than 60 mEq/L **should not** be given in peripheral vein.
- Make sure KCl mixes with the solution thoroughly—invert and agitate the container to ensure mixing.
- Do not add KCl to a hanging container!
- Administer potassium at a rate not to exceed <u>10 to 20 mEq/hr.</u>
- For extreme hypokalemia, rates should be no more than 40 mEq/h while ECG is monitored.
- KCl administered into the subcutaneous tissue (infiltrated) is extremely irritating and can cause tissue damage. Use extravasation protocol.
- Use infusion pump to control flow rate.
- Use extreme caution for hourly replacement of potassium by secondary infusion.
- Potassium is primarily excreted through the kidneys—check kidney function!

C = COMPATIBLE
N = NOT COMPATIBLE
BLANK = NO DATA AVAILABLE

	Acyclovir Sodium	Amikacin Sulfate	Amphotericin B	Amphotericin B Cholesterol	Ampicillin Sodium	Ampicillin Na/ Sulbactam Na	Atropine Sulfate	Aztreonam	Bumetanide	Butorphanol Tartrate	Cefazolin Sodium
Aminophylline		C			C	N				N	N
Amiodarone HCl		C	C				N	C		N	N
Calcium Chloride		C			N	N					
Calcium Gluconate		C			N	N			C		C
Diltiazem HCl	N	C	C			N	N		C	C	C
Dobutamine HCl	N	C			N			C	C	N	
Dopamine HCl	N		N		N	N		C			
Fentanyl Citrate						C		C			C
Furosemide		N			C						
Heparin Sodium	C	N	C		N	C					C
Hydromorphone	C	C			N		C	C		C	C
Inamrinone Lactate							C				
Insulin, Regular						C	C		C	C	
Lidocaine HCl		C			N						
Lorazepam	C	C				C	C		N	C	
Magnesium Sulfate	C	C	N		N	C			C		C
Meperidine HCl	N	C			N		C	C	C	C	C
Midazolam		C			N	N		C		N	C
Morphine Sulfate	N	C			N	C	C	C		C	C
Nitroglycerin					C						
Nitroprusside Sodium											
Norepinephrine Bitartrate		C				N		N			
Oxytocin		C				C					C
Sodium Bicarbonate	C	C		N			N	C			C
Vasopressin											

C = COMPATIBLE
N = NOT COMPATIBLE
BLANK = NO DATA AVAILABLE

Drug	Chlorthiazide	Chlorpromazine HCl	Cefuroxime Sodium	Ceftriaxone Sodium	Ceftizoxime Sodium	Ceftazidime	Cefoxitin Sodium	Cefotetan Disodium	Cefotaxime Sodium	Cefoperazone Sodium	Cefepine HCl
Aminophylline		N	C	N		N		C	N	C	N
Amiodarone HCl			N	N	N	N					
Calcium Chloride											
Calcium Gluconate											
Diltiazem HCl								C		N	
Dobutamine HCl										N	
Dopamine HCl								C			
Fentanyl Citrate		C							C		
Furosemide								C		C	
Heparin Sodium		C	C	C		N		N			
Hydromorphone		C	C		C		C		C	N	
Inamrinone Lactate											
Insulin, Regular	N							C			
Lidocaine HCL		C		C	C			C			
Lorazepam									C		
Magnesium Sulfate		N						C	C	C	
Meperidine HCl		C	C	C	C	C	C	C	C	N	
Midazolam			N			N			N		
Morphine Sulfate	N	N	C	C	C	C	C	C	C		
Nitroglycerin											
Nitroprusside Sodium											
Norepinephrine Bitartrate	N										
Oxytocin		C						C	C	C	
Sodium Bicarbonate		N			N						
Vasopressin											

COMPAT

C = COMPATIBLE
N = NOT COMPATIBLE
BLANK = NO DATA AVAILABLE

	Ciprofloxacin	Clindamycin Phosphate	Co-Trimoxazole	Dexamethasone	Diazepam	Digoxin	Diltiazem HCl	Diphenhydramine HCI	Doxycycline Hyclate	Droperidol	Drotrecogin Alfa
Vasopressin						C					
Sodium Bicarbonate	N				N		N		N		
Oxytocin		C	C		N					C	
Norepinephrine Bitartrate					N						
Nitroprusside Sodium							C	C			N
Nitroglycerin							C	C			
Morphine Sulfate		C	C	C		C			C	C	
Midazolam	C	C	N	C		C				C	N
Meperidine HCl		C	C	C	N	C	C		C	C	C
Magnesium Sulfate	N	C	C						C		N
Lorazepam	C			C	N			N			
Lidocaine HCl	C			C	N	C	C		C	C	
Insulin, Regular						N	N		C		N
Inamrinone Lactate						C					
Hydromorphone		C	C	N					C	C	
Heparin Sodium	N	C		C							
Furosemide	N				N		N	N		N	N
Fentanyl Citrate		C		C		C					
Dopamine HCl	C						C		N		
Dobutamine HCl	C				N	N	C			N	N
Diltiazem HCl			C			C			C		
Calcium Gluconate	C	N		C					C		
Calcium Chloride											
Amiodarone HCl	C	C				N			C		N
Aminophylline	N	N		C		C	N		C	N	

Glycopyrrolate	Gentamicin Sulfate	Gatifloxacin	Furosemide	Fluconazole	Filgrastim	Fentanyl Citrate	Famotidine	Erythromycin Lactobionate	Erythromycin Gluceptate	Enalaprilat	C = COMPATIBLE N = NOT COMPATIBLE BLANK = NO DATA AVAILABLE
	C	C	C	C	C		C	C	N	C	**Aminophylline**
	C		N	C		C	C	C			**Amiodarone HCl**
		C									**Calcium Chloride**
		C	N	C	C	C			C	C	**Calcium Gluconate**
	C		N	C		C	C			C	**Diltiazem HCl**
		C	N	C		C	C			C	**Dobutamine HCl**
	N	C		C		C	C			C	**Dopamine HCl**
	C	C	C							C	**Fentanyl Citrate**
	N	N	C	N	N	C	N				**Furosemide**
				N			N		C		**Heparin Sodium**
C	C	C			C	C	C	C			**Hydromorphone**
		N						C			**Inamrinone Lactate**
	C							C			**Insulin, Regular**
C		C				C	C			C	**Lidocaine HCL**
	C	C	C	C	C	C	C	C			**Lorazepam**
	C	C				C	C			C	**Magnesium Sulfate**
C	C	C	N	C	C		C	C			**Meperidine HCl**
C	C	C	C		C		C	C			**Midazolam**
C	C	C	N	C	C		C	C		C	**Morphine Sulfate**
		C	N	C			C	C			**Nitroglycerin**
			C					C		C	**Nitroprusside Sodium**
								C			**Norepinephrine Bitartrate**
	C								C		**Oxytocin**
N		C	C		C	C	C	C		C	**Sodium Bicarbonate**
											Vasopressin

COMPAT

C = COMPATIBLE N = NOT COMPATIBLE BLANK = NO DATA AVAILABLE	Granisetron HCl	Haloperidol	Heparin Sodium	Hydralazine HCl	Hydrocortisone	Hydromorphone HCl	Imipenem/Cilastatin	Insulin, Regular	Ketorolac	Labetalol HCl	Levofloxacin
Aminophylline	C		C	N	C			N		C	C
Amiodarone HCl							N	C		C	C
Calcium Chloride					C						
Calcium Gluconate	C		C		N					C	
Diltiazem HCl			N		N		C	N		C	
Dobutamine HCl	C	C	N	C				N		C	C
Dopamine HCl	C	C	C		C			N		C	C
Fentanyl Citrate			C		C	C					
Furosemide	C		C	N	C					N	N
Heparin Sodium				C							
Hydromorphone	C	N	N							N	
Inamrinone Lactate					C						
Insulin, Regular			C		C	C	C			N	N
Lidocaine HCl		C	C		C			C		C	C
Lorazepam	C	C	C		C	C	N		C		C
Magnesium Sulfate		N	C	N	C	C		C		C	
Meperidine HCl	C		C		C		N	C	C	C	
Midazolam		C	C		N	C	N	C		C	
Morphine Sulfate	C	N	C		C			C	C	C	C
Nitroglycerin		C	N	N				C		C	N
Nitroprusside Sodium		N	C					C		C	N
Norepinephrine Bitartrate		C	N		C			N		C	
Oxytocin			C		C			C			
Sodium Bicarbonate	C		C		C	N		C		N	C
Vasopressin			C								

Midazolam HCl	Mezlocillin Sodium	Metronidazole HCl	Metoprolol Tartrate	Metoclopramide HCl	Methylprednisolone	Methicillin Sodium	Meperidine HCl	Mannitol	Lorazepam	Linezolid	C = COMPATIBLE N = NOT COMPATIBLE BLANK = NO DATA AVAILABLE
		C		C	N	N	N			C	**Aminophylline**
C	N	C			C				C		**Amiodarone HCl**
						N					**Calcium Chloride**
C				N	C	C					**Calcium Gluconate**
							C		C		**Diltiazem HCl**
N							C			C	**Dobutamine HCl**
C		N			C		C	C		C	**Dopamine HCl**
C		C							C	C	**Fentanyl Citrate**
N				N			N	N	C	C	**Furosemide**
		C									**Heparin Sodium**
C	C	C							C	C	**Hydromorphone**
					C						**Inamrinone Lactate**
C				C			C				**Insulin, Regular**
				C	N		C			C	**Lidocaine HCL**
		C		N					C	C	**Lorazepam**
		C		C			C			C	**Magnesium Sulfate**
C	N	C	C		C	N	C			C	**Meperidine HCl**
C		C				N	C			C	**Midazolam**
C	C	C	C	C	C	N	N			C	**Morphine Sulfate**
C										C	**Nitroglycerin**
C											**Nitroprusside Sodium**
C					C	N					**Norepinephrine Bitartrate**
		C					C				**Oxytocin**
N				N			C	N	C	C	**Sodium Bicarbonate**
											Vasopressin

COMPAT

COMPAT

C = COMPATIBLE
N = NOT COMPATIBLE
BLANK = NO DATA AVAILABLE

	Minocycline HCl	Morphine Sulfate	Nafcillin Sodium	Nalbuphine HCl	Ondansetron HCl	Oxacillin Sodium	Pantoprazole	Penicillin G Potassium	Phenobarbital Sodium	Phenylephrine HCl	Phenytoin
Vasopressin										C	
Sodium Bicarbonate		C	C	N	N			N	N		
Oxytocin		C	C			C		C			
Norepinephrine Bitartrate		C	N			N		N	N	C	N
Nitroprusside Sodium		C									
Nitroglycerin											N
Morphine Sulfate	N	C	N		C	C		C	N		N
Midazolam		C	N	C	C						
Meperidine HCl	N	N	N		C	C		C	N		N
Magnesium Sulfate	C	C	C		C	C		N			
Lorazepam		C			N						
Lidocaine HCL		C	C					C		C	N
Insulin, Regular		C	C					N	N		N
Inamrinone Lactate										C	
Hydromorphone	N		N		C	C		C			
Heparin Sodium										C	
Furosemide		N			N						
Fentanyl Citrate			C								
Dopamine HCl		C	C		C	C		C			
Dobutamine HCl		C	N							C	
Diltiazem HCl						C		C			N
Calcium Gluconate						N		C	C	C	N
Calcium Chloride		C	C					C	C	C	
Amiodarone HCl		C	C					C		C	
Aminophylline		C	N		N	N		C		C	N

C = COMPATIBLE
N = NOT COMPATIBLE
BLANK = NO DATA AVAILABLE

	Verapamil HCl	Vancomycin HCl	Tobramycin Sulfate	Ticarcillin/Clavulanate	Ticarcillin Disodium	Sodium Bicarbonate	Promethazine HCl	Prochlorperazine	Prednisolone	Piperacillin/Tazobactam	Piperacillin Sodium
Aminophylline	N	N				C	N	N	C	C	N
Amiodarone HCl	C	C	C				N			N	N
Calcium Chloride		C	N				N		N		
Calcium Gluconate	C	C	C				N	N	N		C
Diltiazem HCl		C	C	C	C		N				C
Dobutamine HCl	C						N	C		N	
Dopamine HCl		C	C				C				
Fentanyl Citrate	C		C				C				
Furosemide	C		C				C	N			C
Heparin Sodium											
Hydromorphone	C	C	C		C	N	C	N		C	C
Inamrinone Lactate							C				
Insulin, Regular	C	C	C	C	C	C					
Lidocaine HCL	C								C		C
Lorazepam		C								C	C
Magnesium Sulfate	C	C	C		C	N	C		N	C	C
Meperidine HCl	C	C	C	C	C	N	C	C		C	C
Midazolam		C	C				N	C			C
Morphine Sulfate	C	C	C	C	C	C	C	N		C	C
Nitroglycerin	C										
Nitroprusside Sodium	C										
Norepinephrine Bitartrate	C						N		C		
Oxytocin	C	C	C		C				N		C
Sodium Bicarbonate	C	N					C	N		C	C
Vasopressin	C										

New studies may alter the information on all the preceding charts. Adapted from Phillips LD. IV Therapy Notes: Nurse's Clinical Pocket Guide. FA Davis Company. Philadelphia. 2005.

COMPAT

COMPAT

Illustration Credits

Photographs on pp. 30, 32, and 33 courtesy of Bill Ennis.

References

Josephson DL. Intravenous Infusion Therapy for Nurses, 2nd ed. Thomson: Delmar Learning. New York. 2004.

Lilley L, Harrington S, Snyder J. Pharmacology and the Nursing Process, 4th ed. Mosby (Elsevier). St. Louis. 2005.

Myers E. LPN Notes: Nurse's Clinical Pocket Guide. FA Davis Company. Philadelphia. 2004.

Myers E. RNotes: Nurse's Clinical Pocket Guide, 2nd ed. FA Davis Company. Philadelphia. 2006.

Phillips LD. IV Therapy Notes: Nurse's Clinical Pocket Guide. FA Davis Company. Philadelphia. 2005.

Notes

COMPAT

Notes

Notes

Notes

Notes

168

Notes

MRC BOOKSTORE
TOMLINSON
IV MED NOTES (COIL BOUND) /
NURSE.REF   010

9780803614468
1008 $24.95 CDN